THE FEMALE STRESS SYNDROME

How to recognize and live with it

Georgia Witkin-Lanoil, Ph.D.

BERKLEY BOOKS, NEW YORK

This Berkley book contains the complete
text of the original hardcover edition.

THE FEMALE STRESS SYNDROME:
HOW TO RECOGNIZE AND LIVE WITH IT

A Berkley Book / published by arrangement with
Newmarket Press

PRINTING HISTORY
Newmarket Press edition published 1984
Berkley edition / May 1985

ISBN: 0-425-10295-5

A BERKLEY BOOK ® TM 757,375
Berkley Books are published by The Berkley Publishing Group,
200 Madison Avenue, New York, NY 10016.
The name "BERKLEY" and the "B" logo
are trademarks belonging to Berkley Publishing Corporation.

PRINTED IN THE UNITED STATES OF AMERICA

10   9   8   7   6

TO
my mother and father,
my loving family,
and my dear friends,

> *with special thanks to*
> *Esther Margolis*
> *Larry Abrams*
> *Constance Freeman*
> *Joseph Hankin*
> *Jerry Bucci*
> *Patricia Schreiner-Engel*
> *Raul C. Schiavi*
> *Sharon B. Diamond*
> *Katherine Heintzelman*
> *and my wonderful daughter,*
> *Kimberly Hope*

Contents

Foreword

As a psychiatrist who specializes in both couple therapy and sex therapy, and (not incidentally) as a man, I found myself so involved with this book, so impressed with its relevance to my clinical work, that I started making a mental list of people to whom I wanted to recommend it. The first three on the list were all men —husbands I see together with their wives for couple psychotherapy.

Dr. Witkin-Lanoil's absorbing, sympathetic discussion of the constantly shifting biological stress and conflicting cultural pressures that women face—subjecting them to stress symptoms over and above the more publicized ones that all of us, being human, must bear—is important for women *and* for the men in their lives. A woman will come away from reading *The Female Stress Syndrome* with a greater understanding and respect for her own feelings and moods, and a more complete and realistic idea of her options for dealing with stress. A man reading this book will also gain knowledge, of course, but more important he will gain *empathy*; he should come a lot closer to understanding what it must feel like to be female in this culture and time.

As a book written primarily for general readers, rather than professionals, it is I believe unprecedented in scope: it collects important findings from endocrinology, physiology, developmental psychology, anthropology, medicine, and clinical psychology into a single readable, even gripping account of how gender-linked stresses, biological and cultural, can interact to shape and sometimes distort women's health, marriages, and careers. The brief clinical case examples, many of which are drawn from Dr. Witkin-Lanoil's own psychotherapy practice, are simple, clear, and well-chosen. Because they are also so unmistakably human, they help crystallize the problems outlined in the text.

The advice that Dr. Witkin-Lanoil gives about how to deal specifically with stresses and symptoms is safe, practical, and very useful. Undoubtedly, some women will have difficulty implementing some of the important elements of a stress-management program on their own, particularly when they are mired in stress stemming from relationships. Their partners may actively oppose or undermine their efforts to make changes, and/or the women themselves may retain certain blind spots about their own contributions to a troubled union. In these cases—as with those who suffer from acute severe depression or recurrent panic

attacks, and those whose problems are medically com-
plicated—professional help should also be sought, as
is indicated throughout the book.

Dr. Witkin-Lanoil's description of the female reproductive cycle and its hypothalmic/hormonal control, including information on premenstrual tension,
amenorrhea, and menopause, is one of the most lucid,
easy-to-understand accounts I've ever read. For this
reason alone her book should be welcomed by family
doctors, internists, obstetricians, gynecologists, psychologists, and psychiatrists who are looking for a
summary of these processes that their patients can
readily understand. Women who are concerned about
their health and who want to know themselves better
will find much here of great benefit; I applaud Dr.
Witkin-Lanoil for her important contribution in writing this very informative book.

Lee Birk, M.D.
Clinical Director, Learning Therapies, Inc.
Associate Clinical Professor of Psychiatry,
Harvard Medical School

Introduction

We are warned every day about the potential dangers of stress. We are told that stress can be held responsible for high blood pressure and low blood pressure; for overeating and loss of appetite; for fatigue and for hyperactivity; for talkativeness and for withdrawal; for hot flashes and for cold chills. We are advised that under stress we are more susceptible to infection, depression, accidents, viruses, colds, heart attacks, and even cancer. We worry about the aging effects of stress and then worry about the effects of worrying! We are stress-conscious and stress-concerned. We are not, however, sufficiently stress-educated.

Our stress education is inadequate because its main focus has been on men and their life-work patterns. Executive pressures, corporate games, professional expectations, Type A behaviors, and competitive behaviors have been described by the experts mainly with men in mind. For years newspapers, books, magazines, television specials, and lecturers have discussed the serious effects of stress on men—high blood pressure and heart problems, in particular.

But women, after all, live in the same world as men. They both get cut off in traffic, hassled at work, and disappointed in love. They both worry about their families, become frightened by the future, and are surprised by the present.

Women become depressed, unable to sleep, withdrawn, irritable, childish, frightened, anxious, listless, and distracted under stress, just like men. Under stress, women can lose interest in food, sex, or friends, just like men. Their blood pressure may climb, their heart rate may double, their breathing may become fast and irregular, their hands and feet may become cold and clammy, their mouth may become dry and their digestion may seem to stop altogether—just like men.

In addition, women experience some stresses all their own. Men do not menstruate, become pregnant, or go through menopause. Men do not typically have to justify their marital status to an employer or their sexual behavior to their family. Women must deal continually with society's mixed messages: they are most often expected to be sexy, but not sexual; to have a child, but remain childlike; to be assertive, but not aggressive; to hold a job, but not neglect their home. Etcetera.

These special, all-female stresses—both physiological and psychological—result in many symptoms of tension that are unique to women, and many others that are found more frequently in women than in men

—symptoms ranging from loss of menstruation to crippling panic attacks; from transient headaches to life-threatening anorexia. And yet when women complain of these symptoms of tension and stress, they tend not to be taken as seriously as men are. Whereas men are given serious tests and treatment for their ailments, many physicians still prescribe tranquilizers for women, or tell them, "Go home and try to relax. Your problem is just stress."

"Just stress." I am always amazed when I hear that phrase. "Just stress" can trigger or contribute to diabetes, hypertension, and heart attacks. "Just stress" can trigger or contribute to depression, anxiety, insomnia, accidents, alcoholism, and drug abuse. "Just stress" can mimic senility, mental retardation, hyperactivity, and motor coordination problems. "Just stress" mediates all psychosomatic disorders, including ulcers, asthma, and allergies. And "just stress" can bring on the cluster of psychological and physiological symptoms women suffer that I have come to call the Female Stress Syndrome.

My awareness of the Female Stress Syndrome did not, as you might imagine, come from a recognition of my own stresses and stress symptoms. I was as much a victim of female stress unawareness as were my female psychotherapy patients. I was a full-time college professor, full-time psychotherapist, full-time mother, full-time author of textbooks, part-time clinical supervisor, part-time consultant, semi-efficient homemaker, and inefficient bookkeeper.

I was full-time stressed and part-time guilt-ridden. Like most working mothers, I was haunted by a long list of *shoulds*. I *should* be more active in the PTA. I *should* be baking or building with my daughter on snowy afternoons. I *should* be editing or billing *instead* of baking with my daughter on a snowy afternoon! Like most women, I was concerned with the shape of my body and wardrobe—or the lack thereof. Like most homeowners, I was plagued with put-off repairs and immediate emergencies. Like most people in their middle years, I was worrying about time running faster than I could.

Symptoms? Of course I had symptoms. Headaches, backaches, erratic premenstrual tension, unusual allergies, a touch of colitis, and a bit of cardiac arrhythmia. "Just stress," my doctor said. "Just stress," I reassured myself, and continued on my harried way.

Ironically, my Female Stress Syndrome awareness was first raised by a man, who was telling me about his daughter. She had a new marriage, new house, new baby, and a full-blown stress syndrome. She was very unhappy, and feeling very guilty about being unhappy. "I'd be overwhelmed by all that change and responsibility," he said, "but *she* thinks that she should be able to do everything and bake bread, too. Please tell her as a psychologist, woman-to-woman, that it's OK for her to feel stressed. That she can sympathize with herself and help herself without feeling guilty or inadequate. No one else is telling her that!" "Of course I'll speak to her," I replied; and I began to think about the many stresses that fall primarily on women.

My second consciousness-raising experience followed the next week. I was leading a stress-management workshop. Because it was sponsored by a hospital, rather than a police department or corporation, the audience had more women than usual. I was fascinated. I gradually realized that the questions and concerns expressed by the women were different than those raised by the men. The women spoke of many more stresses that were long-term and largely beyond their control—the two factors that make stress dangerous to psychological and physical health! They spoke of unequal pay and unequal say. They spoke of double duties: housework and work-work. They spoke of sabotage on the home front: sometimes intentional, but more often not. And they kept adding, "No one takes me seriously until I am sick in bed for a week!"

Sensitized to this issue of women and stress, then, I went over a decade of therapy notes about female patients. What stresses could women claim as their own? I found many:

- The stresses associated with their *physiology*— breast development, menstruation, pregnancy, and menopause.
- The stresses that can be associated with their *life changes*—becoming a wife, becoming a mother, being either during the divorce boom and economic bust, being female after forty in a youth-beauty culture, becoming a not-so-merry widow, or reorganizing after children have grown.
- The *psychological* stresses often felt by the supposedly swinging single who was raised in an old-fashioned way, the homemaker who is pressured to get out of the home and develop herself, the career woman who is pressured to get back into her home lest she lose her family, and the life-long nonassertiveness expert.
- The *hidden stresses* that distract, distress, and deplete—tokenism, chauvinism, subtle sexism practiced by both men and other women, enter-

taining, chauffering, and talking to two-year-olds.

- And the stresses of *life crises*, which fall largely on female shoulders—caring for an ill or dying parent, parenting a handicapped child, and making sure that life goes on.

Like the stresses mentioned by the women attending my workshop, these stresses are also long-term and beyond immediate control. Like the women at the workshop, my patients felt the symptoms of stress, but were not taken seriously. Their husbands, doctors, and even their mothers too often said, "Get a good night's sleep and you'll feel better in the morning." When they didn't feel better in the morning, they sought a therapist and came to me.

I realized, in time, that the way I was able to help them most was to reassure them that their stresses were not "all in their minds," but, rather, in their daily lives; that their symptoms were usually not in their imaginations, but, rather, in their bodies. In effect, I gave them the "permission" they needed to take stress seriously, and encouraged them to educate themselves about their stresses and stress symptoms.

I wrote this book so I could help even more women educate themselves about female stress and the unique ways in which it affects their lives differently than men's, because of biology and conditioning. I hope this book will also help educate the men who are professionally or personally concerned for the women in their lives.

Educating oneself about Female Stress Syndrome symptoms, however, is only half the solution to a healthier life. Unfortunately, many women become expert at identifying and describing their states of tension and symptoms of stress, but don't go beyond that. They find themselves in the same stressful situations again and again. They recognize that they've been there before, but they cannot change their reactions, no matter how upsetting. These women have yet to take the next step, that of stress *management*, which I also emphasize in this book and believe is as important as stress education. To reduce stress and achieve some control over it, we not only need to know and recognize our problems, but we need to gain an understanding of their causes, and learn how to deal with them. I hope this book helps you help yourself live with female stress, so that you can manage it, rather than have it manage you.

1

Good Stress,
Bad Stress,
and Female Stress

Men and women may be created equal, but they are
certainly not identical—particularly when it comes to
stress. Research continues to uncover fascinating differences between most males and females, some of
which are good news for women and their relationship
to stress.

For example, females seem to survive birth stress
better than males. Although 105 males are born for
every 100 females, by the end of one year there is
already a reversal in the male/female ratio. Not only
is the early female mortality rate lower than the male
rate, but females usually live longer as well. U.S.
Census Bureau reports show that there are only 68
men for every 100 women over sixty-five years of age.

By eighty or more years of age, women make up 2.6 percent of the population, and men only 1.5 percent.

Women also seem to grow older more gracefully. They tend to retain use of their legs and hands longer, show less gray hair, fewer sight and hearing deficits, and less memory loss, and maintain greater circulation of blood to the brain.

Karl Pribram, at the University of California at Santa Cruz, is studying the differences between female and male brains. He has found evidence that suggests some more good news—females demonstrate more left-brain-hemisphere dominance than males. The left hemisphere seems to be in charge of language, logic, and labels, and so girls begin to talk earlier and find school subjects such as English and literature easier than boys do. They may also handle stress more logically and verbally than will boys.

Furthermore, Pribram suggests, the band of nerve fibers that connects the two hemispheres of the brain is thicker in most females. This would give females a greater use of *both* hemispheres than males. That is, females seem to combine the right-brain visual spatial abilities with the left-brain verbal skills in a coordinated way, instead of favoring one hemisphere. (Could this be a scientific explanation of female intuition?)

Since women typically have a greater fat-to-muscle ratio than men, they have better protection from the cold, better buoyancy in water, and a slower release of energy supply. This is a boon to women who are long-distance runners or long-distance swimmers. It also helps women cope with long-term stress, since stress tends to constrict the surface blood vessels that keep our hands and feet warm; stress tends to increase sweating, which chills us; and stress tends to suppress appetite, which makes it necessary to have an alternate source of energy.

From Eleanor Maccoby at Stanford University comes the news that females probably react to touch more easily than males. Might this mean that females get more pleasure from being stroked and caressed than males? Perhaps. Might this mean that females' stress can be soothed more easily by holding, hugging, and touching? Probably!

Some studies show that females are more sensitive to pain than males, other studies show no difference—but *no* studies show males to be more sensitive to pain. How is this good news? Although a low pain threshold may lead to an overconcern with body ailments, it can also provide an early warning system for stress symptoms that require early intervention. This sex difference may even contribute to longer life expectancies for women than for men.

Research also shows a male-female difference in aggression control. After eighteen months of age, girls seem to gain better control over their tempers than boys (E. Maccoby and C. Jacklin°). This is another reason that females could be expected to evolve better verbal stress-coping strategies than less-controlled males. They would assess information more efficiently and address problems more logically. An alternate hypothesis is that females may show less of a tendency to react to situations aggressively and, therefore, need less control. This too would enhance their coping capacity—they would think first, act later.

° For further information on the research and specific studies referred to throughout this book, see the Bibliography beginning on page 201.

One area of female superiority certainly seems underutilized: the female's fine-muscle coordination. Although this would suit women for occupations such as brain surgery and fine art, in this society it more often results in a woman doing needlepoint to reduce tension!

Now for the bad news concerning women in relation to stress. Because of their unique physiology and conditioning, women under long-term stress are in a position of double jeopardy: they are at risk for all the usual stress symptoms, from ulcers to hypertension to chronic fatigue, and they are also at risk for such additional stress-mediated disorders as infertility, premenstrual tension, and anxiety neurosis—a full list of symptoms that are either unique to women or are more frequently reported by women than men. Before detailing these specific female stress symptoms, though, let's first take a look at the general subject of stress and the ways in which the body reacts to it.

STRESS AND THE GENERAL ADAPTATION SYNDROME

Have you noticed how your heart seems to skip a beat or race after a near-accident on the highway? How about an unexpected encounter with a former lover? In each of these instances, your body is responding to signals from your sympathetic nervous system. It can, for example, increase your heart rate from about 70 beats per minute to 140 beats per minute when you are under stress.

Think about your most recent experience with stress. Since this can involve almost any demand or pressure that induced mental or physical tension, an incident will probably come to mind easily. You may remember being upset, frightened, excited, confused, insulted, elated, aroused, disappointed, annoyed, competitive, saddened, sickened, fatigued, exhausted, or surprised.

Stress can result from something happening around us, or from something happening within. It can result from a work problem, a family crisis, or a bout of self-doubt. It can be caused by factors as diverse as the aging of our bodies and the birth of a long-awaited child. It can be intermittent, rapid-fire, or chronic.

The primary effect of stress is to mobilize the body's "fight, flight, or fright" system. This means that stress stimulates the chemical, physical, and psychological changes that prepare us to cope with a threatening situation in these ways. This is all very well, of course, when the stressful situation calls for this type of action; we can easily speculate, for example, that the system evolved back when the "fight" impulse was directed toward defending one's territory or competing for a mate; when "flight" generally meant running for one's life from a wild animal; and when "fright" referred to confrontation with a natural disaster.

Suppose, though—as happens all too often in modern life—that the stress you are confronted with does *not* require action. Suppose, for example, that you are late for an important appointment and are held up in bumper-to-bumper traffic. No movement, no escape, and no action. In this situation, relaxation would be of more use than the biochemical and psychological changes created by the fight, flight, or fright system.

As Hans Selye pointed out in the 1950s, our stress mobilization system is relatively nonspecific. That is, it mobilizes in a similar way to *any* strong demand, whether short-term or long-term; whether it requires action or restricts action; whether it brings good news or bad news. Winning a lottery, for example, stresses the body in much the same way as *losing* a lottery does! Both produce what Selye called the General Adaptation Syndrome—a bodily reaction to stressful situations that involves emergency activation of both the nervous system and the endocrine (hormonal) system.

Within the nervous system, stress messages travel along three pathways. They travel from the brain through motor nerves to arm, leg, and other skeletal muscles, preparing them for motion. They travel from the brain to the autonomic nervous system, which raises blood pressure, heart rate, and blood sugar level; releases reserve red blood cells needed for carrying oxygen to muscles; and slows intestinal movement (since digestion is not a priority in an emergency). And finally, they travel from the brain to the interior of the adrenal gland, which releases adrenaline into the bloodstream as a general stimulant.

The hypothalamus also receives stress messages transmitted from the brain along nervous system pathways, but from there a second system, the hormonal or endocrine system, is activated. This system works more slowly than the nervous system in reaction to stress, but it can maintain its effects on the body for longer periods of time.

Think of the hypothalamus as the emotion control center of the brain. From the hypothalamus, stress messages can be dispatched to many different glands.

When the pituitary is signaled by the hypothalamus, it releases hormones into the bloodstream, which activate the adrenal cortex. The adrenal cortex releases similar hormones, and together they raise the white blood cell count (affecting some immune and allergic reactions), alter the salt and water balance (gradually increasing blood pressure by changing excretion patterns), and stimulate the thyroid gland (increasing metabolism).

THE EFFECTS OF SHORT- AND LONG-TERM STRESS

Both the immediate action of the nervous system and the time-release action of the endocrine system function to prepare and maintain the body for life-saving action. If stress is short-term, there is usually no problem, since your body will have time to rest afterward. This occurs naturally when stress is part of a game, a sport, or even romance. The exhilarating feeling you get is "good stress," stemming from activities that are stimulating and can be terminated at will.

If, however, the stress is long-term and *beyond your control*, your body will not have a chance to rest. The effects of this "bad stress" may begin to show. Your heart, after all, is a muscle, not a perpetual-motion machine. Soon you may feel missed beats, rapid beats (tachycardia), a sense of pounding, or even chest pains.

Breathing patterns also change under stress. Breathing becomes more rapid, often doubling its rate, and it also becomes more shallow, like panting. Under "good" stress these changes are adaptive.

Under long-term or "bad" stress, they create problems. The nose and mouth begin to feel dry from rapid, shallow breathing, and, again, chest pains may develop from working the diaphragm muscles so hard.

Since signals to breathe come from a buildup of carbon dioxide in the bloodstream, rapid, shallow breathing can create another problem: carbon dioxide is expelled *too* well and breathing messages seem to slow down. We feel out of breath and dizzy. This is called hyperventilation, a common symptom of prolonged stress. For quick relief of hyperventilation, you can breathe into and out of a paper bag. In this way, carbon dioxide that has been expelled is breathed into the lungs again, and the carbon dioxide level in the bloodstream is soon high enough to trigger the breathing reflex.

Some psychosomatic effects of "bad" stress are more difficult to manage than hyperventilation. Decreased rhythmic contractions of the digestive system and vasoconstriction of the gastric glands under stress can produce an upset stomach and constipation. (On a trip, we usually blame these symptoms on the water.) The output of certain hormones (glucocorticoids) under stress can gradually increase stomach acidity and, therefore, the risk of a peptic ulcer.

Long-term stress can also produce a *progression* of side effects. The General Adaptation Syndrome, for example, shifts blood flow to large skeletal muscles and decreases flow to the gastrointestinal tract and to the skin. The first signs of such shifts might be cold hands and feet, then gradually a pale or sallow complexion, and finally migraine headaches or high blood pressure.

As another example, the endocrine glands under long-term stress cause the release of extra sugars for energy into the bloodstream, and extra insulin to break down these sugars for use. If too much insulin is produced, blood sugar levels will become too low (a condition called hypoglycemia). We feel tired and reach for a cigarette, coffee, cola, or sweets to give us a lift. Then even more insulin production is stimulated, and the low-blood-sugar cycle continues.

Sometimes long-term stress aggravates a preexisting condition or tendency. Think of this type of stress side-effect as wear and tear on the body's weak spots. Researchers A. H. Schmale and H. P. Iker think that 80 percent of *all* diseases can be explained this way!

Look at the list of stress-related problems below. How many have you noticed in yourself? Your family? Your friends?

ulcerative colitis	cardiac arrhythmia
peptic ulcer	hyperventilation
irritable bowel	asthma
syndrome	rheumatoid arthritis
myocardial infarction	allergies
(heart attack)	skin disorders
essential hypertension	
(high blood pressure)	

Sometimes the symptoms of stress are less serious than these but mimic serious diseases. This, of course, adds further worry to any stressful situation. I often hear patients in the midst of emotional traumas conclude that they have a brain tumor, coronary disease, or cancer, based on some of the stress symptoms listed on the next page.

headaches	dizziness
swallowing difficulties (esophageal spasms)	chest pains
	backaches
heartburn (hyperacidity)	urinary frequency
	muscle spasms
nausea	memory impairment
stomach "knots" or "butterflies"	panic attacks
	constipation
cold sweats	diarrhea
neck aches	insomnia
chronic fatigue	

We know that the brain plays a crucial role in determining how the body reacts to stress. Here are the three important mind-body connections:

1. Remember those stress messages that travel from the brain through motor nerves to arm, leg, and other skeletal muscles? Their short-term effect is to prepare us for emergencies. Their long-term effect is to fatigue those muscles and produce symptoms.

2. Other stress messages travel from the brain through autonomic nerves to the heart, lungs, intestines, sweat glands, blood vessels, liver, kidneys, endocrine glands, and other organs. Their short-term effect is to gear up the fight, flight, or fright system. Their long-term effect is to exhaust these organs.

3. Finally, some stress messages travel from the hypothalamus in the brain to the pituitary and then to other glands that will release hormones. The short-term effect of these hormones is to raise energy production. The long-term effect

is often to create imbalances—and nowhere is this more apparent than in the problems that develop in the woman's finely tuned reproductive system.

FEMALE STRESS

The stress symptoms I've been talking about can and do affect men and women equally; but, as I noted earlier, women are at risk not only for these ailments but *also* for less well-understood symptoms stemming from their particular physiology, life changes, and the social and psychological demands placed upon them. Most important, the majority of these stresses are long-term and beyond their control—the most dangerous type of stress one can experience. Stress-mediated symptoms that are unique to women include

amenorrhea (loss of menstruation)	vaginismus (painful intercourse)
premenstrual tension/ headache complex	frigidity (inhibited sexual arousal)
postpartum depression	anorgasm
menopausal melancholia	infertility

Disorders that are *not* unique to women, but are reported more frequently by them, include

anorexia	anxiety neurosis
bulimia	depressive psychosis

These are the symptoms of the Female Stress Syndrome, and the sooner we make the connection between their appearance and the incidence of stress in our daily lives, the sooner we can help ourselves become healthier. Some women may already have recognized the importance of the mind-body connection by observing their own physical reactions when they are under chronic stress. Many have probably not recognized it, however, and will be relieved to be able to identify both female stresses and female stress symptoms. Remember, the stresses and symptoms of the Female Stress Syndrome do not replace, but rather coexist with, the general stresses and stress symptoms of everyday life. In the next two chapters, we will examine the effects of this double dose of stress on the female body.

2

Stress and the Female Body

Women are endowed by nature with three complex physiological processes that have no counterpart in men: menstruation, pregnancy, and menopause. These changes are all aspects of a very precious gift, of course—the ability to reproduce—but they can also be both the cause of and the arena for a unique set of stress-related problems. Again, we see how important the mind-body connection is in the development of the Female Stress Syndrome.

THE RISK OF PREMENSTRUAL TENSION/HEADACHE COMPLEX

Research has recently begun to document what women have always known: premenstrual tension is real! During the seven to fourteen days preceding menstruation (and sometimes during or immediately after menstruation), its symptoms can include

headaches
anxiety and nervousness
fatigue
depression and/or crying jags
moodiness (alternating highs and lows)
backache and/or pelvic pain
fluid retention and bloating
food cravings (typically candy, cake, and chocolate)
sweating
swelling of the legs
distended stomach with or without stomach upset
irritability
breast engorgement and tenderness
temperature changes
migraine
lowered sex drive
increase in accidents and errors
acne, blotching
flaring of allergic reactions
outbursts of aggression

Quite a list! It is because these symptoms are so extensive that, until quite recently, many physicians dismissed premenstrual tension as an imaginary condition that gave women a good excuse for not coping with their daily lives. How could such different kinds of symptoms (and seventy-five others not listed) be related?

Nevertheless, research over the past twenty years shows that, indeed, more than half the surveyed female populations in three countries (United States, Britain, and France) report psychological and/or physical menstrual changes. In fact, they are probably suffering from different subtypes of premenstrual tension. Katharina Dalton, the British physician who specializes in this area, found correlations between the premenstrual phase and commission of violent crimes, death from accidents, death from suicide, and admissions to psychiatric hospitals among women. L. Rees reports a correlation between anxiety and the premenstrual phase. M. Abramson and J. R. Torghele found headaches to be the most frequently reported premenstrual symptom; and Gail Keith of the University of Illinois Medical Center finds that a sense of being out of control is the most frequent symptom.

Doris's case is not unique. She reports:

> I begin to become short-tempered and irritable as I get closer to my period—irritable in every way. I can't tolerate the noise, the heat, or my children's bickering. I can't even tolerate being touched or stroked. I find excuses to be angry at my family so I can self-righteously go off by myself for a while. Then there is my headache. It comes three days before my period and lasts for two! Aside from eating chocolate and sleeping, the world seems to be empty of pleasure.

Can Doris's problems be explained? Why do headaches develop premenstrually? Why do women become bloated? Tense? Depressed? Why do they become sugar-starved and feel like the Wicked Witch of the West?

Although psychological explanations sound good, they do not fit all of the data. For example, many women who do not suffer from premenstrual tension grew up with the same negative messages about menstruation as the women who do. Many women develop premenstrual symptoms only after the birth of their first child. Furthermore, women who are not ovulating *rarely* have premenstrual stress symptoms.

The triggers, therefore, are probably within the body. The menstrual cycle is highly complex and powerful, involving the monthly gearing up of the entire reproductive system. Because it is an endocrine/hormone-activated system, its hormones travel in the bloodstream as do the stress hormones, thus reaching every tissue in the body. Also, like the stress hormones, the menstrual hormones set off various chemical reactions and metabolic changes in addition to reaching their target organs.

The cycle is governed by those two master glands, the hypothalamus and the pituitary. In the normal cycle, the hypothalamus signals the pituitary to release follicle-stimulating hormone (FSH), which causes several egg follicles in the ovaries to begin growing and secreting the first of the major female hormones, estrogen.

This powerful hormone begins changing the body to prepare for the fertilization of an egg. It causes the cells in the uterine lining to multiply and increases their blood supply. It works changes on the fallopian tubes and on the musculature of the uterus, the cervix, and the vagina.

In addition to these changes in the reproductive organs, estrogen affects the duct system in the breasts; the hormones from the thyroid and adrenal glands and the pancreas; the blood vessels; the chemistry of cholesterol and protein in the blood; and bone metabolism.

After nine or ten days, the high estrogen level in the blood triggers the hypothalamus to signal the pituitary to decrease its FSH output and release luteinizing hormone (LH). This induces ovulation from one egg follicle and a subsequent surge of the second female hormone, progesterone, from the follicle (now referred to as the corpus luteum).

Progesterone, interestingly, *opposes* estrogen—that is, it has an inhibiting or reversing effect on the changes estrogen has produced. (This is one reason why many doctors, such as Penny Wise Budoff, believe estrogen replacement alone for menopausal women can cause problems—the effects of estrogen are not balanced by progesterone as they are normally in the menstruating woman.)

Progesterone stops the growth of the uterine lining and further develops it to receive a fertilized egg. If the egg is fertilized and implants in the uterus, progesterone will continue to be secreted to support the egg's environment until the placenta takes over that function. Progesterone also begins reversing the changes in the uterus, cervix, and fallopian tubes.

Although the level of estrogen has gradually fallen as that of progesterone has risen, on about the twenty-first day of the cycle both are at high levels—and for many women, so is tension! Then if no pregnancy occurs, both hormones are abruptly shut off by the endocrine system's negative feedback mechanism: the high levels of progesterone signal the hypothalamus to stop the pituitary's secretion of LH, which in turn stops the ovaries from secreting progesterone and estrogen.

As the uterine lining breaks down and flows out, both hormones are at their lowest ebb. But the lack of progesterone then induces the hypothalamus to again signal the pituitary to release FSH, starting a new cycle.

As you can see, if one part of this cycle is altered, the rest will also be affected. Thus, there are many possibilities for sources of premenstrual tension.

1. One researcher, Katharina Dalton, has suggested that there is some evidence that progesterone may be involved, since it is often deficient among women with premenstrual tension/ headache complex.

2. Research currently suggests that the estrogen-progesterone ratio may be a factor. When estrogen is too high or progesterone levels too low in relation to each other, symptoms seem to develop.

3. Since hormone imbalances and diet changes can affect water retention and electrolyte concentrations, this area is also being researched. In 1971 psychologist Karen Paige conducted a study in which the hormone levels in a group of women were kept constant by using artificial hormones. She found *no* mood shifts for anxiety and hostility during their monthly cycles!

4. Fluctuations in chemicals involved in brain activity are being examined for sensitivity to estrogen and progesterone changes.

5. Rather than changes in actual hormone levels, changes in some women's *sensitivity* to hormones may explain premenstrual symptoms.

6. There may be withdrawal reactions to the hormones when they decrease just before the menstrual flow.

7. Changes in the way vitamin B_6 is utilized in the body premenstrually may lead to an increase

in a hormone called prolactin. Prolactin in turn can affect fluid retention, causing breast tenderness, swelling, and irritability.

8. Prolactin may also decrease levels of a brain chemical called serotonin, and this may encourage depression, food cravings, and mood swings. Watch for further research in this area.

Can stress affect premenstrual tension (PMT) symptoms? Of course! According to gynecologist Sharon Diamond of Mount Sinai Medical College, stress influences the brain's hypothalamus, which in turn mediates the anterior pituitary and, therefore, the ovaries, the source of the progesterone and estrogen involved in PMT. Stress will aggravate most PMT symptoms from acne to allergies. It aggravates the premenstrual symptoms of temperature changes and sweating. It alters tolerance for fatigue, aches, pains, and other people. In other words, premenstrual symptoms will certainly feel worse, and even *be* worse, when a woman is under stress. If she must deal with skepticism about PMT and lack of sympathy as well —more stress!

Fortunately, both medical science and home science have at least partial remedies for PMT. Physicians have recently begun to prescribe antiprostaglandins to counteract premenstrual and menstrual cramping. Tranquilizers can be prescribed for mood changes, but in this case, awareness that mood changes are temporary and follow a premenstrual pattern may be just as effective—without the side effects of tranquilizers.

Home remedies include cutting back on salt intake to reduce water retention (don't overdo this in the summer), heating pads to reduce the discomfort of cramping in the pelvis and/or back, and, under medical supervision, taking low doses of vitamin B_6 daily beginning ten days before menstruation to counteract possible deficiencies. Since PMT can contribute to the Female Stress Syndrome and vice versa, all the self-help and stress-management techniques that are described in later chapters of this book may well make an important difference. Try them this month—if not for your sake, for the sake of those around you.

THE STRESS RISKS
INVOLVED IN PREGNANCY

Pregnancy means change, and the stress of change often brings on female stress symptoms. If you are a mother, think of all that changed for you during pregnancy. Most obvious, of course, was the change in your body and perhaps your assessment of your attractiveness. Your health-care responsibilities broadened and alcohol, nicotine, and medication intake had to be monitored.

Your activity level probably changed as a result of morning sickness, which 70 percent of women experience as their estrogen level climbs. If your mate told you that your morning sickness was "in your head" and you *knew* that it was in your stomach, further stress was obviously added to an already unhappy situation. Your activity level may have slowed even more as your size and weight increased, but soon after delivery you came to suspect that you might never have a moment to sit still again.

Remember, too, how many financial changes were taking place: impending medical and hospital bills, perhaps the end of your wage-earning for a while, or the beginning of life insurance and saving deposits. And these expenses were just the beginning!

Women often find that their time frame changes during pregnancy. For many women, all plans become focused on the due date, and all experiences are remembered as being far from, or close to, delivery. It is even more important to an understanding of the Female Stress Syndrome to realize that many women do not have clear plans or expectations beyond that date.

Women may have studied reproduction in biology class, genetics and conception in anatomy and physiology courses, natural childbirth methods in Lamaze classes, gentle birth in LeBoyer's books, and neonatal care in maternity classes—but most have never studied mothering! Expectations of motherhood are often no closer to reality than a cartoon is to life; the demands and disappointments this can lead to contribute to the Female Stress Syndrome.

Premotherhood

Premotherhood is a psychological period, not a time period. It may begin before conception, during pregnancy, or even after the onset of labor! Tension can build, drain energy from happy anticipation, and aggravate postpartum Female Stress Syndrome symptoms.

The cases of Sarah, Edna, and Sandy reflect some of the stresses that can be associated with conception.

Sarah had been working as a production assistant in a Chicago advertising agency, dating Ray, and feeling good about her self-directed life-style. Although she stated that in principle birth control was the responsibility of both members of a couple, she preferred the sexual spontaneity that an intrauterine device gave her to the "clumsiness" of a condom. Since she had, therefore, taken on the responsibility of contraception, she was particularly stressed when she accidentally conceived. Although she decided that she wanted the child, she found that she was upset about having lost control over this area of her life decisions, resentful of the changes that were coming, and guilty about her resentment.

Stress for Sarah, therefore, began during premotherhood when she experienced a dip in the predictability of her life. Her pregnancy represented both a wish and a fear, and such ambivalent feelings are always associated with some degree of discomfort or stress.

Although Edna's pregnancy was unplanned, it was a welcome surprise. Edna had worried that she and her husband were not ready for parenthood, that they had more "playing" to do before settling down to the responsibilities of a family. She also suspected, however, that they might never feel ready to make a conscious decision about having a baby, and might delay such a decision far too long. So she put her concerns aside, and prepared for delivery with great excitement. As the time for delivery loomed, however, the realities of parenthood began to frighten Edna and her husband. They became irritable with each other, and each began to see the other as responsible for their plight.

For Edna, stress had begun to build as she approached delivery. She felt that her course was set, that she no longer had a choice about parenting, and that she had betrayed herself by leaving the conception of her child to chance.

> Sandy pondered the considerations of timing, finances, and emotional readiness before she and her husband tried to conceive a child. When the situation seemed right, Sandy was ready. Unfortunately, almost 15 percent of all pregnancies end in miscarriage or spontaneous abortion before the eighth week, and this was Sandy's experience. Following her miscarriage, Sandy's efforts to conceive again were unsuccessful for many months. By the time she did conceive, her anxiety level was high and her focus on motherhood was all-consuming. Even her relationship to her husband was overshadowed by the prospect of the mother-child relationship to come.

Fear and unrealistic expectations combined to produce a high level of stress for Sandy during her pregnancy. Again, motherhood stress began during premotherhood.

Sandy, Edna, and Sarah are by no means unusual cases—their stories are representative of many women's. Premotherhood concerns are a very real part of the Female Stress Syndrome. Some pregnancy fears are symptomatic of a generalized anxiety about the demands that are made on mothers, as in the case of Edna. Other fears, however, are probably literal—fear of miscarriage, of having a defective baby, of labor pain, or even of delivery procedures or cesarian section. Either way, motherhood becomes associated with fear.

Postpartum Depression

Depending on the particular study you read, between 20 and 65 percent of childbearing women report maternity blues. Since postpartum (after-the-birth) depression rarely begins before the third day after delivery, it seems clear that hormonal and chemical changes are involved. But psychological stresses also play an important role.

Psychologically stressful changes begin with delivery. The woman is separated from her husband and family except during visiting hours. She is often separated from her baby except during feeding hours. Soon the new mother feels isolated, vulnerable, and incapacitated. Her first days at home with the baby can make things worse. Mary remembers:

I was totally prepared for natural childbirth, and totally unprepared for natural child-rearing. Despite my twenty years of formal education, I did not know how to sterilize a bottle without melting the rubber nipples. By the end of the week, every time my baby cried, I cried, too.

Teenage mothers struggle with further stresses after delivery. Becoming a mother may have solved an identity crisis, but it also may have created new ones: loss of freedom, of mobility, and of choice, and mixed feelings about parenting and its responsibilities.

Some women don't feel the baby blues until they have their second or third child. As Dora, who has four children, put it, "It is hard to see myself as pretty, witty, and wise, when I feel more like the old woman who lived in a shoe, and had so many children that she didn't know what to do!"

The postpartum depression should lift as the new mother rejoins her support system, sees that she can handle things, and finds that her body chemistry readjusts. Sometimes it does not. As with some other Female Stress Syndrome symptoms, professional intervention may be necessary to break the mind-body chain of events producing, in this case, the depression.

THE STRESS RISKS INVOLVED IN MENOPAUSE

Even the most skeptical of physicians and mates usually view menopausal depression as "real." That is, they assume *physiological* changes within the woman can explain mood and behavior changes. She is more likely to receive sympathy and understanding at this time than when she is premenstrual or going through a postpartum depression.

Who can argue with the reality of the hot flashes that the majority of menopausal women experience? Who can argue with the reality of the permanent cessation of menstruation that results from the end of ovarian activity? These symptoms are neither imaginary nor psychosomatic in origin, all agree; therefore, menopause must be real.

The sympathy doesn't stop here. Physicians and husbands understand that menopause represents a landmark along the road to aging. Who can argue with the assumption that a woman will be depressed at the notion of aging? Who can argue with the idea that the loss of fertility makes a woman naturally defensive and irritable? Who can argue with the belief that when a woman feels older her sex drive decreases? Researchers can—and do.

It is ironic that much of this sympathy is unnecessary and may even be unhealthy: unnecessary because the most recent research points out that most women do *not* experience increased depression or any other type of mental illness during menopause (S. McKinlay and M. Jeffreys, 1974, for example); unhealthy because such sympathy may encourage women to feel defensive and devalued by assuming that they *should* feel that way during and after menopause.

The happy truth is that many women find the freedom from fear of pregnancy liberating, both sexually and practically. With menopause comes a rite of passage into a period of personal choice and self-defined life-styles—free from premenstrual tension and postpartum blues, free from preparental anxiety, and filled with postparental relaxation.

According to Lena, now sixty-two years old, the fun has just begun. At thirty-eight she started to plan for her retirement from mothering. She enrolled in a counseling program that had evening classes. By the time Lena reached menopause, she had completed her master's degree in social work, completed her full-time mothering responsibilities, and completed her ten-year plan to prepare for her second career. It has been five years since she began private practice, and she is pleased that she sorted her interests sequentially, rather than juggling them simultaneously.

Of course, this is not to say that menopause is always a time free from sadness and stress. Even in women who look forward to their life changes, there may be nostalgia for earlier times, a sense of loss of their ability to have children, and an anxiety associated with entering a later stage of life. Furthermore, menopause is a time of major physical change. Life change and physical change interact, once again. Female stress symptoms can appear, once again.

Physical Changes

Like the General Adaptation Syndrome itself, menopause affects nearly every organ in the body.

It begins gradually as the number of egg-containing follicles in the ovaries is reduced, so that the amount of estrogen produced when the pituitary sends out FSH falls below normal levels. Eventually the delicate hormonal feedback system is disrupted. The pituitary sends out more and more FSH and LH, because not enough estrogen and progesterone are coming from the ovaries to shut them off.

The high levels of FSH seem to make the follicles develop more rapidly, thus shortening the cycle by a couple of days. A follicle in a given cycle may not ovulate or form a corpus luteum, and without the proper amount of progesterone from this phase of the cycle, the uterine lining thickens without maturing properly. As a result, it may slough off in bits and pieces, causing spotting. When so little estrogen is produced that the uterine lining does not build up enough to flow at all, menstruation ceases.

Not surprisingly, the withdrawal of estrogen and

progesterone from tissues that had been flooded with them monthly has its effects. Blood chemistry and blood vessels must adjust to the change. The adjustment of the vascular system to the loss of estrogen is thought to cause the hot flashes that are experienced by two-thirds of menopausal women (it has been shown in research studies that the flashes cease if estrogen is replaced). The vaginal and urinary tract tissues tend to become dry and thin and thus more vulnerable to infections. Sometimes painful intercourse and urinary problems result.

Bone metabolism loses an important support with the withdrawal of estrogen and progesterone. Everyone, including men, loses bone mass with aging, but postmenopausal women lose it at a higher-than-normal rate. In fact, osteoporosis—bones made brittle by loss of minerals—will probably occur in about 40 percent of all women.

Finally, some women do experience anxiety and depression that seem to be related to the reduction of hormone levels—just as premenstrual and postpartum emotional effects can be.

Individual Differences

As in all aspects of the Female Stress Syndrome, individual differences are important determinants of symptoms. L. Speroff, R. H. Glass, and N. G. Kase have summarized the influences on the average woman's menopausal pattern.

1. *Rate of hormonal changes.* Usually, menopausal changes begin a few years before menstruation actually ceases, and the body has time to make

a natural transition by approximately forty-eight, the national mean age for menopausal women. If this is the case, brief hot flashes and amenorrhea (cessation of menstruation) may be the only symptoms of menopause. Most women who experience hot flashes have them for about a year, although some women report ten years of these vascular changes. If, however, the hormone feedback to the hypothalamus is withdrawn suddenly, as with a total hysterectomy including removal of the ovaries, menopausal symptoms may be more severe and numerous. "Instant menopause" can produce instant symptoms: fatigue, insomnia, heart palpitations, back pain, and moodiness. In addition, any surgery can produce anxiety; surgical removal of reproductive organs can result in a profound sense of loss as well. Since messages of anxiety and loss can affect hormonal functioning through the complex hypothalamus connection, both "instant" and natural menopause symptoms will be aggravated by stress.

2. *Amount of hormone depletion.* Estrogen levels gradually drop as the ovaries become less active. Since the changes in the vaginal wall and the autonomic nervous system are related to estrogen depletion, symptoms of menopause such as dyspareunia (pain during intercourse), diminished vaginal lubrication, and hot flashes will be more severe among women who have greater estrogen depletion. Although estrogen-progesterone-replacement therapy may relieve these symptoms, the elevated risk for certain medical conditions means that it is not always recom-

mended. Water-soluble jellies can relieve vaginal dryness with less risk, and a fan and a sense of humor may help make hot flashes bearable.

3. *Physical fitness.* Although menopause has genetic parameters, nurture also has an influence. Hormonal changes can lower resistance to infection by changing the acid/alkaline balance in the vagina and urethra; nutrition and exercise can help to restore resistance. Changes in calcium and fat metabolism are part of menopause; exercise and nutrition can help to compensate for some of the effects of these changes. In fact, as nutrition and vitamin awareness has improved over the years, the average age of menopause onset has been set back and menstruation onset has been set forward!

4. *The meaning of aging.* As with all mind-body syndromes, menopause has an autonomic nervous system component, a hormonal component, and a cerebral cortex (brain) component, with the hypothalamus as the information-processing and control center. If the thought of aging is distressful, this message will go from the brain to the hypothalamus to the autonomic and hormonal systems; and the General Adaptation Syndrome will gear up for a long-term stress situation. With menopausal changes also affecting these mechanisms, a woman may experience a *multiplication* of the symptoms of both stress and menopause. If, in addition, the symptoms themselves make her more anxious, we see a vicious cycle in which more autonomic changes lead to more hot flashes, and so on.

Many times of body change are times of stress, because we may feel our sense of control threatened. The changes associated with menopause, as with menstruation and pregnancy, are preprogrammed; we can make them better or worse, but we can't turn them off! This may increase anxiety and make many women feel helpless or victimized by their bodies.

> Marilyn had always exercised, dieted, and maintained a youthful style of dress. She felt that her appearance and health were in her own hands and that her self-discipline was the secret of her "staying power." Although she thought that she had accepted the inevitability of menopause, she found that when menopausal changes began, her sense of control was threatened. She looked for, and of course found, every new wrinkle and age spot that appeared. She could no longer predict the rate of her body's changes, and her stress level rose. Feeling that she was fighting a losing battle, she lost her interest in dieting, exercise, and dressing attractively. She became increasingly depressed; soon Female Stress Syndrome symptoms, which she blamed on menopause, developed.

Does Marilyn's story sound familiar? Although the menopausal symptoms themselves may not be under full control, other areas of functioning are. Unlike Marilyn, women who maintain control of their weight, their exercise, and their time can help themselves reduce that feeling of being overwhelmed by inevitable physical changes. Take appropriate control over every area that you can while you are menopausal, and see Chapter 9 for more on the management of menopausal stress.

Depression and stress are not exclusive to changes in body state such as menstruation, pregnancy, and menopause. In fact, often these feelings coincide with body changes only because both come at the same time of life, not because one has been *caused* by the other. For example, a husband's retirement, a daughter's failing marriage, or the loss of one's own parent may trigger a depression mistakenly labeled "menopausal melancholia." The loss of one's office friends or autonomy may coincide with the post-partum period. To understand the Female Stress Syndrome fully, we must look in the next chapter at stresses not associated with preprogrammed body changes, and at the body changes that go along with these stresses.

Female Stress Symptoms

Some of these symptoms of stress are common; some are less so. Some are unique to women; some are simply found more frequently in women than in men. Some involve a physical predisposition; others do not. They are all important aspects of the Female Stress Syndrome.

ANOREXIA NERVOSA

Donna cuts her food into many little pieces and moves them around her plate. She drinks her coffee and eats the lettuce in her salad, but will not swallow the meat she has put in her mouth. She coughs into her napkin to remove it. Donna is twenty years old, five feet four inches tall, and weighs eighty-seven pounds. Although she has abundant energy for physical activities, within two weeks her malnutrition will endanger her life. Even then she will not seek help voluntarily. She feels fat and wants no interference with her dieting.

Donna's syndrome is called anorexia nervosa, and it is one of the many stress-related symptoms that are more frequently found among women than among men.

Under the stress of increasingly adult responsibilities, sexual anxiety, or self-conscious concern about their appearance, young women may begin to control their eating and thereby gain a sense of control over their other impulses as well. Soon their appetite is altered, but their body image is not. As young women like Donna become more and more emaciated, their self-image lags behind, and they continue to see themselves as needing to diet.

Why is this disorder so much more common among women than among men? The answer is not clear, but it probably involves female physiology. Appetite changes often accompany the menstrual cycle, for example. Premenstrual cravings for sugars, chocolate, and rich or spicy foods are common. The food preferences that accompany pregnancy are legendary. (Pickles and ice cream, anyone?)

Even if women were not more physiologically predisposed to anorexia nervosa, cultural messages probably encourage women to manage stress symbolically through anorexia.

Cindy was the oldest of many children and felt like a surrogate mother to her brothers and sisters. A little more was always expected of her, and she tried her best to live up to all expectations. Her grades were excellent, her friends were "nice," and her family was proud. By the time she was a high-school senior, Cindy was anorexic.

If Cindy is thought of as having "swallowed" others' demands all her life, the stage is set for her not "swallowing" any more. By late adolescence, she was facing additional adult responsibilities. Not the openly defiant type to begin with, Cindy took control over herself in this passive way. Her rebellion was symbolic.

> Theresa seemed to be using her anorexia to manage sexual anxieties. She actually delayed her own sexual development by keeping her body thin and childlike. Since her fat/muscle ratio was altered by dieting, even her menstruation was delayed. She dispelled her guilt over sexual impulses by denying her "appetites," and her fantasy fear of pregnancy was dispelled by a perpetually flat belly.

Although her mother thought Theresa would be tired from her constant dieting, she found instead that her daughter was overactive. Psychologists would suspect that Theresa's hyperactivity was yet one more attempt to manage unacceptable impulses, by keeping very busy.

There is no mystery as to how anorexia nervosa reflects an obsessional concern with appearance. Anorexics are often "approval junkies," trying to live on love and acceptance rather than food. If thin is in, they will want to be the thinnest. If fat means a lack of willpower, they will avoid being fat at all costs: by starvation, vomiting, enemas, and diuretics, to name a few.

At what point should family members worry about a dieting young woman? As soon as they see her dieting excessively without medical supervision, becoming obsessed with fasts, water diets, or fad-food diets. As soon as they suspect her body image is unrealistic. As soon as dieting interferes with her normal menstrual cycle. As soon as they find evidence of her using forced vomiting, enemas, or diuretics to control weight gain. Psychotherapy, family therapy, group therapy, and even hypnotherapy can all help if the problem is treated early enough. If allowed to become severe, anorexia is life-threatening. In fact, some reports say that up to 15 percent of severe anorexia patients die of malnutrition or related complications.

BULIMIA

How many women are thinking, despite these gloomy statistics, that they would gladly trade in their compulsive eating for a "mild case" of anorexia? Undoubtedly more women feed themselves than starve themselves when they are under stress. They chomp, chew, and sip, trying to sweeten up, spice up, or fill up their lives.

When gorging and binging become extreme and compulsive, the resulting stress symptom is called bulimia. Its source can vary, since food can have many different correspondences and meanings. Food can be tied to a memory of being mothered. It can provide a touch of home. It can be a reward, or it can be part of an attempt to gain strength and fortification. It can be a substitute for "taking in" sexual pleasure, praise, or love from others. It can be a safe outlet for anger: we can chew it, bite it, or cut it. It can be a safe outlet for dependency needs: we can hide it, stock it, and hoard it. The list may go on and on, but the symptom remains the same—uncontrolled eating.

> Gloria binged secretly. Publicly she complained that her sluggish metabolism was responsible for her weight. Privately, she used her obesity as an excuse for her lack of popularity. She periodically tried to diet, but felt too deprived to continue for long. When she was tense, she could imagine no other release, and told herself that her eating was a combination of a bad habit and good cooking.

Gloria was a food addict, and as with other dependencies, management of her symptom would be a lifelong problem. First she would have to recognize that she was no longer a helpless infant whose only active capacity for soothing herself was to put something in her mouth. She would have to understand that when she had finished her munching, the source of her stress had still not been dealt with! She would have to admit to bulimia. The stress triggers would have to be identified and alternative strategies for coping developed.

Bulimics run many of the same health risks as anorexics. Their diet becomes nutritionally unbalanced as they "just pick" at healthful foods to compensate for devouring desserts or junk food. Their biochemical electrolyte balance becomes threatened if they use forced vomiting, enemas, and/or diuretics to undo their loss of eating control. If they hide their bulimia by maintaining normal weight, the disorder is harder to identify and help is less likely to be offered. If they alternate between anorexia and bulimia, they are in double jeopardy.

ALCOHOLISM

Statistics tell us that male alcoholics outnumber female alcoholics almost five to one in the United States, but, for several reasons, this probably does not accurately reflect the incidence of alcoholism among women. In fact, the ratio is changing. As greater numbers of women are working outside the home, their alcohol problems are becoming more obvious. As women deal with the stresses of what used to be a "man's world," their alcohol problems increase. Not surprisingly, so do those of homemakers who feel less and less support for their chosen role. More and more, women are seeking treatment for drinking problems. So, while alcoholism is not a distinctively female stress symptom, women must recognize it as an important potential response to stress.

Alcohol can act as both a sedative and a disinhibitor. Both functions can temporarily reduce a sense of stress. As a sedative, alcohol works like a liquid barbituate. At low levels it slows muscle response and induces a feeling of relaxation. As a disinhibitor, it affects the brain center for emotional behavior and allows the drinker to act out impulses with less guilt. The effect will vary depending upon which of the drinker's impulses are more guilt-associated. If, for example, it is your aggressive impulses that make you feel most guilty and stressed, a few cocktails may transform you into a woman who speaks her mind without hesitation. A few more and you may be speaking without consideration, fore-thought, or discretion, as well. If, on the other hand, it is your sexual impulses that are ordinarily repressed, you might find yourself dancing on the piano after a few drinks. A stoic may become a crying drinker; an "earthmother" type may become a teenager reborn.

The problem with this elixir of relaxation and disinhibition is that moderation is difficult. Since the effects of alcohol are achieved by altering judgment, alcohol abuse is difficult to avoid. If one drink makes us feel good, we reason, two drinks will make us feel better. Right? Actually, as alcohol consumption increases, motor coordination is impaired, drowsiness progresses into drunkenness, and memory is diminished. We eventually sleep, but dreaming is suppressed and our intestines are affected. The day after is rarely worth the night before. Stresses have not been altered, and in addition our capacity to deal with them has been lowered.

At what point does alcohol use become alcohol abuse? The following brief summary is drawn from the definitions set forth by the World Health Organization, the *Comprehensive Textbook of Psychiatry* (Second Edition), and Alcoholics Anonymous.

1. Frequent intoxication or drunkenness (four times per year or more).
2. Habitual use (drinks at dinner having an effect more than once a week).
3. Compulsive drinking (without real choice or control, or out of fear of not being armed with a drink).

4. Addiction (characterized by withdrawal symptoms, such as tremors, seizures, disorientation, or hallucinations).
5. Vocational, social, or physical impairment related to alcohol consumption.

When signs like these are present, the drinker is confronted with two problems: the original stresses and the alcohol abuse they have triggered. Both problems must be treated, and professional help is usually vital. Group therapy, family therapy, or individual therapy, with a trained psychiatrist, psychologist, social worker, nurse, or Alcoholics Anonymous leader all seem to work if the patient is motivated and the therapist is supportive and caring.

HEADACHES

If headache jokes were fact, it would seem that migraines occur exclusively among long-married women when they are approached sexually by their husbands. Although this is not true, migraines *are* more frequently a female than a male stress symptom. The question is, why?

It would seem that there is a predisposition to react to stress in this way built in to the female physiology. Glands, various blood vessels, and scalp muscles may, under the influence of some female hormones, be particularly susceptible to stress triggers. Blood vessels that constrict spasmodically in reaction to stress may eventually dilate painfully. The walls of the vessels are now irritated and the blood pulsing through feels like pounding pain. This type of headache is a true migraine. Prolonged contraction of the muscles of the face, neck, and scalp produces what is generally called a tension headache. And, finally, secretions from various glands to raise energy levels under stress can also change fluid retention and electrolyte balances, causing yet a third type of headache.

Although fast relief from headache pain is offered in myriad television commercials, relief from the stresses that cause migraine headaches is even better.

> Rosemary knew that her migraine attacks always followed situations in which she was enraged but felt that she couldn't express her anger. She claimed that she had had years of "nonassertiveness training," and feared that showing her anger would destroy her image as the patient wife and mother. She was, in fact, quite sure that her husband would stop loving her if he knew how often she felt irritable and annoyed at being taken for granted.

Imagine Rosemary's surprise when she began to request some appreciation from her family and got it! Her headaches gradually subsided, and she learned that her stress trigger had been an automatic fear of her own angry impulses. Other women have found that their dependency needs or sexual interests create similar conflicts and activate their headaches.

If the "unacceptable" impulse can't be identified or avoided, migraine may warrant a preventive medication (such as methysergide maleate) or ergotamine at its onset. Biofeedback techniques can be effective also, by helping women recognize autonomic nervous system changes *before* they reach headache proportions, and thus modulate fight, flight, or fright responses.

AMENORRHEA

If a girl has not started to menstruate by eighteen years of age, the diagnosis is "primary amenorrhea." If, however, there has been menstruation and it stops, the condition is called "secondary amenorrhea." Although both types of amenorrhea can be related to organic problems, stress is the most frequent cause of secondary amenorrhea.

The mind-body chain of events works like this: stress is perceived and messages are sent through the nervous system to activate the fight, flight, or fright emergency systems. Since the reproductive system is not an emergency support system, its hormone levels are lowered and menstruation is not triggered.

Imagine this: A sexual encounter has caused Sally great anxiety, fear, and guilt. She is distraught at the notion that she may have become pregnant. She worries and worries and waits breathlessly for her period. Her period is delayed by her stress, and her anxiety increases. The scene is set for temporary amenorrhea.

Imagine this: Fran is about to leave home to attend boarding school. She realizes that she will be on her own in a real way for the first time in her life. She is fearful yet determined, nostalgic yet excited, reluctant yet committed. She is experiencing an approach-avoidance conflict. These strong mixed feelings have raised her stress level, and the scene is again set for amenorrhea. "Boarding school amenorrhea," in fact.

Imagine this: Carol has decided to transform herself into a facsimile of a *Vogue* model. She begins to diet drastically. She eliminates desserts. Then breads. Then fats. Then sweets. Her menus have been stripped down to celery and bouillon, and she has been stripped down to skin and bones. She has lost her stomach, her hips, her waist, and her period. Amenorrhea!

Imagine this: It is Lissa's last summer before college. This is her last chance to see if she wants an academic life or the life of a professional dancer. She joins a semiprofessional troupe and starts a round of classes at 6 A.M., rehearsals at 1 P.M., and performances at 7 P.M. She makes more and more demands on her body and is proud of its response. She gains a pirouette and loses a period—then another, and another. Again, amenorrhea.

Imagine the many other stressful situations that can also lead to amenorrhea. Depression, prolonged grief, and unrelieved anxiety can produce the same effects. Although mature women do not typically lose their periods, the menstrual cycles of young women are more vulnerable. In fact, young anorexics are frequently nonmenstruating.

A famous study of women college students shows how responsive the female reproduction system is to psychological and social factors. M. K. McClintock reported that although dorm-mates were menstruating at different times throughout the month when they first arrived at college, by the end of the school year their periods were synchronized far beyond chance or coincidence.

What can be done about amenorrhea? Relief from the stress is often enough, although sometimes a normal cycle returns even while the stress continues. Researchers tell us that some concentration-camp victims who developed amenorrhea when they were first imprisoned began to menstruate once again after a few months of confinement—even though their terrible circumstances had not been altered. Just as psyches can adjust to even the most stressful situations, so too can bodies often gradually adapt to stress and change.

Sometimes this does not happen, however. When stress-triggered amenorrhea continues and a normal cycle does not spontaneously reoccur, a physician should be consulted. Although the problem may not have started with an organic condition, chronic stress may lead to one. The physician may suggest therapy based on hormones or a drug called clomiphene.

The doctor may, however, suggest psychotherapy instead. Psychotherapy can help patients deal with the immediate stress causing the amenorrhea and helps to eliminate the risk of future stress symptoms by encouraging the development of more effective coping strategies for the future. Psychotherapy can also help women explore the cultural messages that make menstruation a high-risk target for the Female Stress Syndrome.

MENSTRUATION AND SOCIETY'S MIXED MESSAGES

For many women, sexual stress reflects negative associations with female body functions. As we have discussed, it is women alone who menstruate, gestate, and lactate. They should feel unique, special, and proud. Instead, they often feel embarrassed, inconvenienced, and inferior. Why?

A look at some common taboos shows how women get the message that being female is a physically and psychologically unhealthy state of being.

> Don't swim during menstruation.
> Don't wash your hair during menstruation, because you will get sick.
> Don't handle flowers during menstruation, because they will wilt.
> Don't get a hair permanent during menstruation, because it will not take.
> Don't have intercourse during menstruation.

Menstruation is particularly singled out for negative attitudes. Just when a young woman is trying to cope with the stresses of adolescence, she begins to menstruate. In some cultures, this is a cause for celebration. In our culture, it must be kept a secret.

Jennifer's first menstruation started while she was at school. At first, she was frightened when she noticed red stains on her underpants when she was changing into her gym clothes. She was twelve and had no sex education at school. Her mother had never spoken to her about menstruation—or about anything else that personal, either. Jennifer had never allowed herself to think about "that part" of her body, nor look at her genitals with a mirror. She had only a vague notion of her sexual anatomy, and wasn't too sure exactly where her vagina was in relation to her urethra.

Jennifer had heard from the boys on her school bus that the first "period" was the bloodiest. Her fear turned to worry. She didn't dare go to gym, leave the locker room, or even get up off the bench. She was trapped. She wondered when the cramps and headaches she had heard about would start. Maybe in a few minutes when the flow really began, she concluded. She was still sitting on the bench, frozen by her anxiety and confusion, when she was rescued by a teacher-in-training.

Advertisements for tampons and sanitary napkins emphasize the need to hide any signs of menstruation, avoid any possibility of an "accident," and forego adjusting one's activities in any way. "No one but you will know," they seem to be saying.

Like Jennifer, many adolescents worry about hiding their secret month after month. They feel odd if they start menstruating early in puberty, they feel odd if they start late, and they feel odd *while* they are menstruating. It's certainly not hard to understand how females can develop negative feelings about a body function referred to as

the curse
being unwell
on the rag
sick time
bleeding
a visiting friend
that time of the month

Once a woman starts associating her vagina with a "curse," it is but a short step to developing self-conscious sexual inhibitions.

FRIGIDITY—INHIBITED SEXUAL AROUSAL

The term "frigid" is outdated, although it used to be quite commonly used. It conjured up images of unfeeling, uncaring, icy-cold women who were rigidly unresponsive to demonstrations of physical affection. In fact, the label was meant to describe a sexual dysfunction in which stress interfered with the swelling and lubrication of the female genitals in response to sexual stimulation—a problem that is now called inhibited sexual arousal.

Does this inhibited response mean the woman has no interest in sex or physical affection? Absolutely not! Often she enjoys the contact and is unaware on a conscious level of the source of her fight, flight, or fright reaction.

> Rhonda had looked forward to her honeymoon as a time of romance and privacy. She had lived at home until her marriage and had "saved herself" for her husband. When the time for lovemaking finally arrived, Rhonda found that "nothing happened." She liked being close with her husband, but couldn't share his sexual excitement. He, in turn, felt like a sexual failure, and soon the stress level climbed.

In sex therapy, Rhonda's stress was traced to her self-conscious fears of loss of control. She was concerned about what reactions were "normal." She was so busy worrying that she could not stop watching herself and abandon herself to the pleasure of the experience with her husband. Learning that flushing, spastic movements, nipple erections, rapid breathing, and utterances are all common relieved much of her stress.

VAGINISMUS

Another less common stress-related sexual problem is vaginismus. Women with vaginismus would like to be able to achieve normal sexual intercourse, but find that involuntary contraction of the muscles surrounding the vagina make penetration painful or impossible.

> Flora told her doctor that she thought she had no vaginal opening. Although she had never examined herself with a mirror, she could not feel an orifice with her finger nor insert a tampon. Her doctor attempted a pelvic exam, but found that although her vulva was normal, Flora's involuntary contractions of the pubococcygeus muscles were so strong that she could not be dilated for an internal examination or a Pap smear.

A number of stresses can be responsible for vaginismus, including fear of pain, fear of pregnancy, fear of intimacy, fear of punishment, fear of intrusion, fear of "contamination," fear of dependency, and fear of rape. Vaginismus is, in fact, very often the product of an early rape—by a stranger, date, husband, or even family member. The contractions that were meant to protect the victim from the stress of unwanted intercourse can remain and prevent desired intercourse.

In cases such as this, both the symptom and the stress need treatment. In her book *The New Sex Therapy*, Helen Kaplan recommends gradual dilation and accommodation of the vagina to the patient's own fingers, in the privacy of her own home. If the inhibition seems unyielding, clinical psychologists and psychiatrists trained as sex therapists can help women deal with the underlying fear and stress.

ORGASM PROBLEMS

Perhaps the most common sexual stress symptom among women is orgasmic dysfunction. The statistics vary, but here are some approximations that give the general picture.

- Five to 15 percent of the female population surveyed reports never having achieved an orgasm. This is called primary orgasmic dysfunction. Most researchers, including William Masters and Virginia Johnson in *Human Sexual Inadequacy*, associate this condition with the stress created by guilt. Sexually repressive backgrounds seem common among those who suffer from it.
- Forty-five to 60 percent of the female population surveyed reports having difficulty achieving orgasm at certain times or with certain partners. This is called situational or secondary orgasmic dysfunction, and is usually related to lack of sexual arousal due to the stress of fights or fears. An orgasm requires an autonomic "letting go" and giving up of control; fights and fears, on the other hand, require "holding on" and a struggle *for* control.

There are many other stresses that can inhibit orgasm. Listen to the women in a Westchester, New York, sex therapy group as they discuss this problem.

"I realized, finally, that I was afraid of looking silly if I had an orgasm with my boyfriend. I didn't know if I would make noise or curl my toes the way I do when I come by masturbating. Then I took a good look at him while he was coming. He became spastic and noisy and I loved it. It made me feel great to be part of that; so I let myself go also—and bingo!"

"You know, I never really *wanted* to let Eric give me an orgasm. I didn't want him to have that kind of power over me—pleasure power."

"Fred criticizes me about everything else, so I expected criticism in bed too. Now it doesn't matter to me any more, because I am not criticizing myself. Now I look at him as if he's crazy when he starts in on me—and he stops! Since I began to feel that I'm supposed to enjoy sex, he has picked up on that idea."

"Believe it or not, I was thirty years old before I tried to masturbate, and I was thirty-three before I had an orgasm. My secret fear was that it would feel so good that I'd never want to do anything else! Like women who can't stop eating or drinking, I was afraid I'd have no control over this. The funny thing is that now I feel the opposite way—since I can give myself an orgasm, I am more relaxed about the whole thing."

Fear of punishment, fear of criticism, fear of abandonment, concern with appearing aggressive or selfish, reluctance to give a partner the power of pleasure, anxiety about religious taboos, misinformation, guilt, anger, and control issues can all raise female stress levels and inhibit the orgasmic response. After all, the center for both stress and sexual stimulation is the mind.

Success rates for the treatment of both primary and secondary orgasmic dysfunctions are usually reported to be as high as 80 percent. However,

J. LoPiccolo, a well-known researcher in human sexuality, reminded sex therapists at Mount Sinai Hospital in New York City that these success rates reflect the achievement of an orgasm through *any* means: genital stimulation, clitoral stimulation, masturbation, and vibration—usually not through intercourse alone. For many women, orgasm through intercourse alone, without direct clitoral stimulation, is improbable. So why fight Mother Nature?

INFERTILITY

The Lerners were anxious to begin a family and tried without success for at least one year. Diagnosed as functionally infertile, Mrs. Lerner became more and more frustrated. She began to feel inadequate and helpless. She turned to the experts, but no organic problems could be found. Her concern with her infertility spread to a concern with abandonment. She felt pressed to take action, to take control.

An adoption seemed to be the next logical step. It restored her sense of decision. It provided her with a new focus of activity. It was a goal that she and her husband could share.

The Lerners did, in fact, adopt a girl and begin to parent together. Within the year, Mrs. Lerner became pregnant!

Most psychologists know couples like the Lerners. How do they explain a case in which the woman seems infertile, though no organic reason presents itself, until *after* she has adopted a child? The answer can lie in the Female Stress Syndrome. Fears and conflicts about mothering can produce stress, which in turn interrupts and alters hormonal functioning, which in turn affects ovulation, which in turn provides a solution to the conflict—no pregnancy. After hidden and unconscious fears are dispelled by parenting the adopted baby, stress is reduced, endocrine functioning returns to normal, and conception is more likely.

Great-grandmothers knew a lot about this Female Stress Syndrome symptom. They knew that tension could create temporary infertility. Their recommendation to a couple like the Lerners would have been, "Take a vacation together." It is still worth a try.

ANXIETY REACTIONS

Sylvia was waiting for a bus at the end of a hot summer day. The buses were full and a crowd of commuters swarmed around her. As bus after bus passed them by, Sylvia began to wonder if she would ever get home. She also began to wonder why her breathing was so very shallow and rapid. She felt as though she would have to monitor each breath or her breathing might stop altogether. Her palms, she noticed, were both cold and clammy, and although the air was muggy she was now shivering slightly. More alarmed than bewildered, she started walking home rather than waiting a minute longer for a less-crowded bus. As she half-ran, half-walked, panic welled up. Her heart pounded and she feared that she would not make it home. Terror seemed to come in waves, each leaving her more exhausted than the last. She reached her door, but found that her hands were shaking so violently she could not use her keys. She stood by her door, desperate. Within minutes, however, the panic subsided, and she entered her apartment shaken and mystified.

Sylvia was suffering from a panic attack. Her fight, flight, or fright reaction seemed to come from nowhere. As in the case of Rosemary's headaches, the stress triggering Sylvia's reaction was also an internal conflict between a wish and a fear. Sylvia wished to break loose at the end of her work day but also feared that impulse. She had never tested the impulse, and had no idea where it would lead her. With professional help she came to accept her impulse and handle it realistically—and her panic attacks subsided.

The female-to-male ratio for anxiety disorders is a disturbing three to two. The reason for this is unclear, but part of it may lie in the way girls are raised in our society. According to J. H. Block's research, fathers in this culture emphasize achievement, self-assertion, aggressiveness, and self-aggrandizement in their sons, but expect their daughters to control these same qualities. Is it any wonder that women think of many of their impulses as "dangerous"? Is it any wonder that women see themselves as more fragile and vulnerable than men?

Anxiety attacks are best treated by professionals—psychiatrists, psychologists, and psychiatric social workers. Before, during, and after treatment, however, support systems are vital. So too is knowledge of crisis-intervention procedures, which can help until a professional is found. Read about these procedures in the last chapter of this book, and help others help themselves.

In addition to acute anxiety attacks, women seem to experience more general anxiety than men. Why? Perhaps it is because women are less likely to respond aggressively to stressful situations. Perhaps it is because women are presented with more anxiety-provoking situations and cultural messages that reduce their sense of control. Perhaps it is because women are more apt to notice and label fight, flight, and fright reactions as "anxiety." Perhaps it is because, until recently, girls and women have had fewer sports outlets for tension than boys and men have had. Perhaps it is because men may be less willing to admit that they are also anxious! Perhaps it is due to all the pressures that make up the Female Stress Syndrome.

WEAK LINKS AND OTHER THEORIES

How is it, you may be wondering, that a particular woman develops a particular stress symptom at a particular time?

One theory is that anxiety and stress aggravate problems that already exist because of our genes, prenatal environment, diet, or earlier diseases, damage, or accidents. These vulnerabilities are the *weak links* —symptoms waiting to happen.

Another, similar, theory hypothesizes that each organ and system has lowered resistance levels when the body is subjected to a high enough degree of anxiety or stress. When this happens, a virus, disease, or disorder is more likely to appear.

A third theory claims that a particular woman will develop a particular symptom because she has been reinforced or rewarded for it.

Every time her husband gave her an angry look, Christine's stomach flip-flopped, her knees felt weak, her hands became clammy, and her heart raced. Without realizing it, she would clutch at her chest and press her hand over her heart. She felt all four symptoms, but her husband was only aware of the last one. His angry look would change to a look of concern whenever her hand flew to her heart, and a particular organ-response was thus reinforced. Soon both Christine and her husband worried about her heart rate when she was under stress.

Perhaps, however, each woman has a unique set of responses to each emotion. Five women could react physiologically with five different response patterns when experiencing similar stress. Each might call her own pattern "anxiety," but the different patterns would, of course, produce different symptoms.

Although there is not much research to support it, there is a theory that the fight, flight, or fright response is *not* as nonspecific as Selye described it. This suggests that there are subtle differences in the body's responses to different kinds of stresses. Fright situations could be stressing different organs or systems than fight situations, and so on. Thus, particular stresses might lead to particular symptoms.

Historically, many theories have tried to associate certain stress symptoms with certain personality profiles. Even Sigmund Freud agreed with this approach. In fact, he thought that both a particular personality profile and a particular stress symptom resulted from the same early childhood experiences. A woman with unfulfilled dependency needs, for example, might show more eating and gastrointestinal disorders than is usual, whereas a woman who has difficulty expressing her anger directly might have a tendency to develop sexual dysfunctions.

Two famous women explain female stress symptoms in yet another way. The psychiatrist Karen

Horney and the anthropologist Margaret Mead both trace particular symptoms back to anxiety-provoking communications from mother to child—subtle messages conveyed during feeding, discipline, and emotional demonstrations.

The psychoanalytic schools would argue that a particular organ in a particular woman is affected at a particular time because it is symbolic of a particular conflict she is experiencing. In the following case history, for example, Robin had both a wish and a fear concerning pregnancy.

> Although she worried that she and her husband were not ready for parenthood and its responsibilities, Robin and her husband decided to try to start their family while he was in the Army and had excellent medical coverage. She became more and more excited about the idea of having a baby, and rationalized that she might never feel ready, so why wait? Soon after the decision, Robin stopped menstruating. At first, she assumed she was pregnant. Later it became clear that she was not. The symptom of amenorrhea (lack of menstruation) under stress conditions relieved her of the conflict by eliminating the fear and making the wish "safe."

Many theories about why women develop the symptoms that they do focus on the importance of individual differences among women under stress. It is as if each has her own threshold for psychosomatic reactions, and her own combination of variables that can push her over that threshold.

- The *amount* of stress needed before a symptom is produced can vary.

- The *number of times* the same or similar stress is experienced may affect women differently.
- The *physical condition* of each woman, and her *emotional state* preceding and during exposure to a stressful situation may influence her threshold.
- The significance of *age* to stress symptoms varies from woman to woman, as does the *readiness* to cope or capitulate.

Every one of these theories attempts to explain why a specific stress symptom appears in a particular woman at a particular time. It is most likely, however, that the factors mentioned are *interacting* to produce the various stress symptoms. As you begin to understand your own stress patterns, bear in mind the multi-faceted nature of the Female Stress Syndrome. You can learn to recognize your own physical and psychological vulnerabilities, your reinforcement history, your areas of conflict, your reaction patterns, and your personality profile. You can sort out the symptoms that have symbolic meanings from those that reflect physiological predispositions; and you can learn to differentiate the symptoms you have learned from those you have inherited.

One of the most alarming aspects of the Female Stress Syndrome is that it starts shaping itself almost immediately after we are born! In the next chapter, we will look at the world into which girls are born and see how the groundwork is laid for future stress patterns.

4

Nonassertiveness Training and the Female Stress Syndrome

It's true that every child is a unique individual. It's true that any individual boy can be calm, quiet, and cuddly, and that any individual girl can be active, acrobatic, and athletic. It's true that people—including baby nurses—cannot accurately guess the sex of a baby when it is wrapped in a yellow blanket. It is also true, however, that raising girls and raising boys is different. Ask any parent! Most will tell you that their experience suggests the following:

- Girls are more compliant than boys—more likely to run errands and help out.
- Girls seem more social and concerned with their appearance.

- Girls, although not passive, seem less aggressive than boys.
- Girls show more anxiety than boys.
- Girls use their intuition more.
- Girls speak and read earlier than boys.
- Girls are more emotional and more responsive to emotions.
- Girls have better fine-motor coordination.

Is this because girls are exhibiting genetic differences in their cognition, their physical capacities, and/or their emotional makeup? Might it be due to socially modeled and behaviorally reinforced differences? Or is it, perhaps, caused by an interaction of both?

Although there can be no clear answers here, most parents will tell you that boys are a handful because

- Boys are more active than girls tend to be.
- Boys stay awake longer.
- Boys take everything apart.
- Boys are harder to keep track of, will roam farther and more often.
- Boys lose their tempers more easily than girls.
- Boys prefer more action and violence and less talking than girls, in books, films, and TV.
- Boys engage in more mock fighting and attacks.

Are boys more mechanical than girls, or is it that their curiosity is channeled into dismantling and reconstructing, while girls' curiosity is not? Are boys more aggressive, or is it that their activity level is channeled into contact sports while girls' is not? Or is it both?

Since the different expectations and perceptions that parents and teachers have of girls and boys strongly affects the messages, rewards, punishments, and models each child receives, the question of nature vs. nurture becomes hard to answer. To further complicate the question, children obviously affect their parents as much as parents affect their children. If parents do, indeed, talk more to girl babies than to boy babies, are they *teaching* girls to be better listeners than boys, or are they *responding* to a sex difference? Let's see what research can tell us.

IT'S A GIRL!

Socialization begins at birth. If girls are generally less assertive than boys, then training must begin early. In fact, the sexual stereotypes believed by the parents of a female child obviously *precede* her birth.

Consider the following statistics. H. Barry, M. Bacon, and I. L. Child, studying 110 cultures, found that 82 percent of the people they polled expected females to be *more nurturing* than males; 87 percent expected females to be *less achieving* than males; and 85 percent expected females to be *less self-reliant* than males! Another research team had similar findings: D. Aberle and K. Naegele concluded from their studies that fathers expect daughters to be pretty, sweet, and fragile, whereas they expect their sons to be aggressive and athletic. Are these valid expectations or self-fulfilling prophecies?

It seems that the way parents see their children is consistent with what they expect to see. In a fascinating study by J. Rubin, F. Provenzano, and Z.

Luria, fathers were asked to rate their newborn children's characteristics, with the following results:

- Fathers of daughters rated their babies softer, finer featured, more awkward, less attentive, more delicate, and weaker than did fathers who rated sons.
- Fathers of sons found them to be firmer, larger featured, better coordinated, more alert, stronger, and harder than did fathers who rated daughters.

The most interesting aspect of this was that the birth lengths, weights, and reflex times for *all* babies in the study were the same!

In another piece of research, J. Meyer and B. Sobieszek showed men videotapes of seventeen-month-old children. When the men were told they were looking at a boy, they were more likely to describe the child as active, alert, and aggressive. When they were told they were looking at a girl, they described the baby as cuddly, passive, and delicate.

From perceiving girls and boys differently according to stereotyped images, it is only a short step for parents to create *different realities* for each sex. Research has shown that

- Most girls are treated more protectively than boys. This logically suggests to girls that they must *need* protection.
- Most girls are complimented on their appearance before any other trait. People exclaim, "What a pretty girl!" but "What a big, strong boy!" This,

of course, conveys to girls that their packaging is very important.

- Most girls are handled with more vocalization than are boys. Michael Lewis found that mothers of twelve-week-old girls speak and respond more to the babbling of their babies than do mothers of sons. F. Rebelsky and C. Hanks found the same was true for fathers! Being verbal, therefore, "works" for girls.

When it comes to nonassertiveness training, women and men—mothers and fathers—seem to work in tandem, perhaps reflecting their own training.

- As mentioned previously, in a cross-cultural study J. H. Block found that fathers emphasized assertion, aggression, achievement, and self-aggrandizement in their sons, while emphasizing *control* of aggression and assertion in their daughters.
- Researchers R. Sears, E. Maccoby, and H. Levin found that mothers of kindergarten children tolerate more aggression toward both parents and peers in their sons than in their daughters.
- Another team of researchers, Lisa A. Serbin and K. Daniel O'Leary, found the same was true with nursery school teachers.

Although it would be unlikely that *some* sex differences were not operating here, the influence of socialization on female behavior comes through loud and clear. Males may indeed have a higher activity level in general, and females may indeed have more verbal facility in general, and prenatal hormonal differences may indeed produce brain-hemisphere-dominance differences, as research suggests; but the *direction* these sex-related differences take is related to the Female Stress Syndrome.

THE HIGH PRICE OF SUGAR AND SPICE

The results of nature and/or nurture are swift. By eighteen months of age, girls already show more control over their tempers than do boys. But this sort of control can have a price.

Anxiety that is not directly related to a specific external cause often stems from fear of one's own unacceptable internal impulses. If girls are treated as though their aggressive, assertive, and achieving impulses are unexpected and even undesirable, we can logically anticipate a high anxiety level in young girls as they struggle to control these natural impulses.

Indeed, girls *do* experience much more anxiety than boys. Shocking confirmation of this can be found in a wide range of studies of different groups (quoted in E. Maccoby). To mention just a few, anxiety scores higher than those of comparable groups of boys were found among

132 nine-year-old French girls
470 girls, both white and black, nine to eleven years old
64 nine-year-old American girls
1,249 high-school-aged girls
2,559 females aged thirteen through adulthood
149 college-aged women

Maccoby also quotes studies indicating that both teacher evaluations and self-reports show girls higher than boys on anxiety scales.

Although self-control can be an important ingredient in the development of mature coping strategies, the repression of strong impulses consumes energy and contributes to frustration, depression, and the Female Stress Syndrome.

In high school, Lea had been a star. She was editor of the school yearbook, president of the Spanish club, and captain of the girl's basketball team. Her friends, parents, and teachers all told her that she was special —hardworking, social, and pretty.

Off went Lea to college, where the entire freshman class, she soon learned, was special! Each member had also been a star. Without social, parental, or teacher feedback, Lea began to lose her confidence and her ability to cope. Once that happened, she felt that she was losing control over her ability to achieve and concentrate. High demands, low control, and no positive reinforcements: stress!

Lea was in and out of the infirmary all that year. She had a free-floating fearfulness and kept pinning her sense that something was wrong on her body. Soon, in fact, she did develop mononucleosis and actually moved into the infirmary. This relieved her anxiety for awhile, since she felt, again, as if she were home and under someone's watchful eye. Her impulses to quit school, be taken care of, or, at the very least, stop putting her energy into trying to be so special, were again safely under control. She had learned to perform for others when she was young, and now was on her own . . . passive and purposeless.

Lea's case is not uncommon. Society sends girls a strong message: "Control yourselves!"

FEAR OF FAILURE VS.
NEED FOR ACHIEVEMENT

Fear of failure, like fear of success, is the legacy of nonassertiveness training. Fear of failure is the result of years of being shamed or teased by boys, brothers, fathers, mothers, or teachers whenever a public performance of athletic, mechanical, or combative prowess was attempted. Fear of success is the result of years of being warned against being "too smart" or "too strong" or "too independent." Where are the role models for strong, assertive women in our culture? Some can be found on the sports pages; there are a handful of world leaders to whom we can look; occasionally one hears about prominent business and professional women, or a barrier-smasher such as astronaut Sally Ride is thrust into public view. But these are the exceptions rather than the rule, and generally a major component of the message we get about them is how *unusual* they are—a mixed message indeed.

Need for achievement, however, is built into all of us. It is an extension of our earliest desires to explore, crawl, walk, and run. It is a reflection of our ability to process information, formulate plans, and solve problems. It is an adult expression of our need to gain some control over our environment and solve some of its problems.

It's not uncommon for women to feel a mixture of fear of failure and need for achievement. The head-on collision between the two is what aggravates the Female Stress Syndrome.

The need for achievement moves women toward their goals. Although this need was not explicit in female role expectations over the past few generations in this country, it existed nonetheless. Middle-class women exhibited it through volunteer and community organization work, through vicarious pride in children's achievements, and through identification with their husbands' careers. Working-class women exercised it through their pride in running their homes, in taking care of their families, and in holding jobs for less than equal pay in order to achieve a higher standard of living. Upper-class women expressed it through attempts to increase the power, prestige, and exclusiveness of the family by doing charity work, making large donations to various causes, and orchestrating social events.

The fear of failure, on the other hand, moves women away from their goals. This fear is fed by many stereotypic female role expectations and myths.

Women are the weaker sex.
Women are too emotional for the business world.
Women will always leave their careers for a man.
Women are less logical than men.

Fear of failure moves women away from their goals by involving them in excessive concern with the opinions of others. Failure then means shame, rather than just personal disappointment. Fear of failure requires constant collecting of excuses and a general defensiveness—both of which drain energy from directly pursuing goals!

The classic ring-toss game has been used to show how fear of failure operates. Subjects could stand anywhere they wanted while tossing the rings over the stake. Some walked right up to the stake. Others backed up to make the challenge more difficult. Researchers found that backing up was characteristic of people with high fear of failure. It was an attempt to provide an excuse in case of failure, under the guise of increasing the value of achievement.

Women with a high fear of failure will constantly handicap themselves and increase their own stress in order to defend themselves against failure with excuses. For example, they may schedule too many things at the same time. Or they may never start a task until the last minute.

Today more and more women *are* expressing their need for achievement. Unfortunately, their fear of failure hangs on from early childhood lessons. The vacillation between moving toward goals and backing off from situations involving the risk of failure creates a great deal of constant stress for the "new woman."

Polly wanted a career in real estate. She entered a training course but stopped short of taking her final exam. Too many demands at home made studying impossible, she said. She pursued her career nonetheless. She applied for jobs in real-estate offices but restricted herself to locations close to her home and to working hours that conformed to her teenaged children's school hours. She landed an apprenticeship, but found that family vacations, entertaining, doctors' appointments, and even volunteer activities interfered with her taking the broker's examination required for advancement. She stayed on, working on salary rather than receiving a broker's commission, talking incessantly about her career frustrations. Should she stay in real estate, handicapped as she thought she was, or move to another field? she asked constantly.

Sometimes women are not fully conscious of their ambivalence and the stress it imposes. Their non-assertiveness training has become so much a part of their way of being and their self-image that they don't even realize they are vacillating. At most, they may wonder why they feel so uncertain most of the time, or why they labor over making decisions.

STRESS AND THE SINGLES SCENE

Talk to a few single career women, and you will probably hear stories similar to Mickie's.

Mickie was single, successful, and sexual. She was twenty-nine years old, however, and beginning to feel alone. Not lonely, she explained; *alone*. She wanted a partner. She wanted to meet a man who could join her and share in her life. Perhaps marry. Perhaps have children.

But Mickie was having a hard time. She found men she could "adopt." Men who would make great "wives." Men who would "take her away from hard work and competition." Men who would "take care" of her. Men who truly believed she wanted to be "dominated." And men who truly believed that she wanted to "mother" them. What she could not find was a man who believed her when she said she wanted a partner.

She was successful and loved her work. This made many men feel competitive. She was sexual and yet discriminating. This made many men feel anxious about "performance." She was mature and intelligent. This made many men feel self-conscious. She was self-supporting and financially secure. This made many men feel inadequate.

Mickie's story has a happy ending. She met a man who enjoyed her just as she had wanted to be enjoyed. Her independence was a bonus to him, not an escape from responsibility and not a threat. They are still living happily ever after, arguing about politics rather than about her achievements.

Not all such stories end so well, however. An achieving woman who harbors both fear of failure and fear of success tends to find herself devastated by male rejection, great or small. She blames herself for unsuccessful affairs. She retreats before her partner can. She "obsesses" so much about past problems and future fantasies that, often, she cannot let things be. She may sabotage the relationships herself in order to explain possible failures or to avoid the responsibility of success.

In fact, the achieving single woman has only two options if she is interested in meeting men, neither of them very satisfactory. First, she can be socially nonassertive: that is, she can wait for men to telephone, ask her out to dinner, or initiate sexual advances. Or she can be socially assertive. That is, she can telephone men, invite them for dinner, and initiate sexual advances. The former option can make women feel powerless and stressed; the latter can make them feel vulnerable and stressed. Either way, they are single and stressed!

RETRAINING YOURSELF

As in other areas of the Female Stress Syndrome, understanding the origins of a particular type of stress is only half the battle. Reducing that stress is the very important other half. If you feel that vacillating between the need for achievement and the fear of failure or fear of success is a long-term, chronic source of tension for you, try to bring the problem under control using these techniques.

1. Gather *information*, rather than opinions, about a problem or situation. This will increase your capacity to assess things realistically, and decrease the anticipatory anxiety you may be feeling. The only important opinion will be your own, after you have processed all the information you can.

2. Similarly, look at all situations involving your goals through *your* eyes only; don't try to see yourself as others see you. Spectatoring (looking at yourself to see if you appear to have failed) will only hamper your ability to pursue goals and will usually produce inaccurate information anyway.

3. Try to experience falling short of a goal as unfortunate, or as a learning experience, or as a disappointment, rather than as a failure. This means you must *describe* your behavior, not judge it.

4. Avoid self-blame at all times. Try your best, but don't put yourself on trial. Be your own defense lawyer—not the lawyer for the prosecution.

5. Be task-oriented rather than a praise addict. Focus on finishing a job, not showing it off, and you will reduce your performance anxiety and fear of failure at the same time.

As you work at overcoming the nonassertiveness training you have had, and the female stress symptoms that accompany that training, it may help to remember that you are something of a role-model pioneer. You are on the forefront of social change, but you are not alone. You will be helping the next generation of women come up with some guidelines to aid them in expressing their own needs for achievement. And you will be helping the next generation of *men* establish more realistic and open-minded expectations for female achievement, as well.

5

Love, Sex, and Marriage Under Stress

Many psychologists and psychiatrists compare the state of being in love to that of temporary psychosis. The "symptoms" are almost equally alarming.

- Reality becomes distorted, and a great deal of time is spent obsessively fantasizing about the future.
- Enormous power is bestowed on the loved one. His phone call can produce joy; his absence can produce anxiety; his approval becomes necessary for self-approval; his disapproval leads to self-blame. If he withdraws, as psychiatrist John Astrachan of Cornell University Medical College explains, we add self-insult to injury by assuming

that he would not have done so if *we* had been more loving and understanding. We cannot proceed with our schedules, our plans, our daily lives until he has phoned, written, or made a date.

- Delusions of his perfection emerge and add to the flavor of insanity. Whatever his actual physical appearance, we imagine that he is the height of attractiveness, irresistible not only to ourselves but to others as well.

- There is often a temporary reemergence of childhood beliefs in magic, fairy godmothers, and happily-ever-afters. Even coincidences take on mystical overtones.

Instead of being alarmed, though, most of us seem to enjoy being in love. We hum songs glorifying it, read stories describing it, see films and television programs centering around it, and spend work and leisure time seeking it. Why?

The most obvious answer is that being in love makes us feel good. It lives up to all the cliches—we feel like we're walking on air, have stars in our eyes, and look younger than springtime. (Not a bad disorder, if you can get it!) Scientists tell us that being infatuated probably stimulates increased production of our bodies' natural pain-killing substances, the endorphins. Poets tell us that being in love stimulates our souls. Women tell me that it stimulates their sense of inner beauty.

Nevertheless, it's also true that long-term relationships—and particularly marriages—create a special set of stresses for women. In fact, given the current divorce rate of 50 percent, we might speculate that one major function of infatuation is to facilitate the otherwise terrifying process of marriage!

Unfortunately, many young women find themselves marrying in order to grow up. Even if she is still daughter, student, or in her late teens, a woman has "adult" status once she is married. She is now a wife. She is Mrs. Somebody. A new name, a new home, and a new adult life. But the teenage wife usually pays a high price for this instant new self-definition. She may bypass the identity confusion of these years, but she can become confused and overwhelmed by the responsibilities of marriage instead.

At first Judy said no to Jack's proposal of marriage. She had wanted more in a husband—more maturity and more security. Jack was not quite tall enough, smart enough, or old enough to suit Judy's fantasies. Even his car was second-hand. But then she began to think about marriage in general rather than marriage to Jack. Married, she would not have to live at home nor ask permission to borrow the car. Married, she could give advice, not receive it. Married, she could dismiss forever the anxiety surrounding dateless weekends. Married, she could have a baby— dress it, take care of it, and show it off. Married, she would no longer feel her own life was second-hand. Judy said yes to Jack.

Judy and Jack eloped. They set up home in a walk-up apartment. Soon Jack quit community college to work as a department-store salesman. Both Judy and Jack wanted more for him, but a baby was on the way, and they needed money. The baby and the baby blues arrived at the same time. Judy was constantly tired and lonely. She longed for the days of dates and romantic detours. She longed for her parents' home and the hot meals that she didn't have to prepare herself. What had she been thinking, she asked herself, when she had said yes to Jack?

Even if Judy had not eloped, stress would probably have developed after she had married. As both statistics and clinicians tell us, the act of marriage generally changes even the longest premarital live-in relationships. The factors that seem to be responsible can be labeled the "four R's."

1. *Regression.* Moving into a marriage may spark new plans for home life, but it also activates memories of our parents' marriage and home. With childhood memories come childhood feelings and behaviors. Since these old behaviors are often more practiced and familiar than new, adult perspectives and behaviors, they may keep popping up when least expected. Husbands become confused with daddies and wives may act like daughters, much to their own horror.

2. *Re-creation.* Women may also find that despite their best intentions they are re-creating and perpetuating stereotypical, sexist behaviors. For example, they may find themselves displaying learned helplessness—imitating dependent behaviors that they observed to have worked for their mothers. They may find that they are suffering from the "Cinderella complex"—waiting for the handsome prince to change their lives from emotional rags to riches. They may be acting out "little woman" passivity—living in fear that they will be deserted if they become their own women. Or they may be slipping into nag-

ging aggressiveness—sounding exactly like the women who most repelled them when they were young.

3. *Reaction.* To their surprise, some women find that they *react* more than they act. That is, they monitor their mate's moods and needs, trying to be perfect for him rather than being themselves. They watch every word to make sure that they are giving appropriate, justified responses. They hesitate to initiate plans, conversations, even sex, to avoid the responsibility that goes with self-assertion: plans may not work, conversations may become arguments, sexual overtures may be rejected. They soon feel like spectators of their own lives, and their sense of control erodes until the Female Stress Syndrome surfaces, inevitably.

4. *Recollection.* Memories that may be confusing, unsettling, or stressful are often locked away through repression—a kind of motivated forgetting. This makes our daily lives easier. Marriage, however, can trigger the reappearance of recollections of our parents' marriage—of scenes, screams, and secrets. This, of course, makes coping more difficult. We may find that we are suffering from nightmares, unpleasant daydreams, mood swings, and a free-floating anxiety.

Fritz Perls, the originator of gestalt therapy, popularized the phrase "here and now," and warned us not to use the present to master the past. He observed that many of us re-create our most upsetting relationships of the past again and again to try to gain mastery of the past situation through the present reenactment. Even if we should gain mastery in the present, however, it would not count because the *original* situation in the past would not have been settled—so we would be bound to set up the challenge once again. If you are having trouble moving out of the past and into the "here and now," try the following:

1. Look for evidence of the "four R's" operating. Acknowledge to yourself which are causing you the most trouble.
2. Raise your awareness of them until you can recognize them as they are actually happening. Recognizing their dynamics after they have played themselves out will enable you to make only apologies, not changes!
3. Remind yourself that your increased awareness will permit you to make behavioral choices. Take yourself off automatic pilot and take control of your interactions.
4. If you find it hard to believe that the present can be different from a replay of your past, just try behaving *as if* the present is different from the past. This will set up a positive, rather than negative, self-fulfilling prophecy! Both you and those around you will have a chance to try new actions and new reactions. You may be contributing to the very outcomes you fear most, simply by *expecting* those outcomes and behaving defensively and dejectedly before the problem has begun.

The "four R's" are not the only sources of relationship stress. Females in this culture are often taught that they are the "weaker sex," but they may be rebelliously uncomfortable with emotional dependency. Since young women are often warned that men might want to use them as sex objects, they may be particularly wary of turning their sexual pleasure over to their partners. Since women in this culture often perceive that they may be traded in for a younger model in later years, they may be particularly focused on security. And since women in this culture are often warned that career is primary and marriage secondary for a man, they may deny feelings of rejection by fortifying themselves with anger and adopting a distant, "I don't care" attitude.

Stress can also stem from a bad meshing of the expectations that a new couple usually brings together. Think of it this way: every relationship involves at least four sets of expectations—the woman's expectations for herself; the woman's expectations for her partner's behavior; the man's expectations for himself; and the man's expectations for his partner's behavior. Since role expectations are learned through imitating behavior that seems to work for others, we imitate those whom we see the most: our parents, our siblings, our teachers, and our friends. Thus most role expectations are learned within one's own family and subculture, and identical matches between both partners' expectations would be rare—even impossible! There must be constant adjustment and communication of expectations in an ongoing relationship. And the stresses do not stop there.

- Add the problem of a woman who cannot meet her *own* learned self-expectations. She is likely to bring guilt, self-blame, and feelings of inadequacy to the relationship.

- Add the problem of multiple role conflicts, particularly prevalent in marriage. That is, a woman often finds that her roles as mother, daughter, and friend conflict with the behaviors expected of a wife.

- Add the problems created as role models keep rapidly changing, as they have in the '70s and '80s. Doris Day has given way to Mary Tyler Moore, and she, in turn, to Sally Ride!

- Add the problems of women who preferred their fathers to their mothers as role models in many areas. Such women are usually well-adjusted, high achievers, but they are unlikely to fit into a conventional role.

- Add the special problems of those women who did not have adequate or acceptable female role models at all. They must discard the old and evolve the new simultaneously!

Unfortunately, there is no second chance at childhood. To make relationships work without excessive stress, we must parent ourselves in those areas where our parents were inadequate. We cannot expect our partners to make up for the past.

Go even one step further to take control over *your* daily life by giving yourself permission to develop your own set of relationship expectations. When you do, be realistic; know both yourself and your mate. We are all package deals! Take the bad with the good, the weaknesses with the strengths—develop roles that take both sides into account. Remember, your rela-

tionship is made up of you and him—nobody else. It
is shaped by who the two of you are, not who you
should be.

MANIPULATION TACTICS

Psychiatrists, psychologists, poets, and philosophers all
agree that loving relationships involve a degree of
"letting go," accepting vulnerability, and sharing control—admitting that you care about and can be
affected by your mate's behavior. But if couples
struggle against dreaded feelings of vulnerability and
struggle for a sense of control, they will create fights
to serve both functions. Through fights they try to
convince themselves that they "don't care," that they
can upset their partner, that they can hurt more than
be hurt. Through fights they avoid close, intimate
moments and warm, caring feelings, which might be
so desperately needed that the thought of losing such
a bond becomes worse than pretending the bond
doesn't exist in the first place!

If the real point of a fight turns out to be reducing the stress of vulnerability and/or loss of control,
rather than solving the issue at hand, one or more
of the following manipulation tactics will appear.
Check yourself on this inventory.

MANIPULATION TACTIC	DEFINITION	YES	NO
Mind-reading	Telling your mate what he thinks or feels, despite his protests to the contrary.		

TACTIC	DEFINITION	YES	NO
Sleuthing	Collecting clues and evidence consistent with your own fears and dire prophecies.		
Grab-bagging	Reaching into the past to grab at insults and injustices you have saved up for fights or flights.		
Name-calling	Teasing and taunting your mate in a way which ensures that anxiety-provoking issues will not get faced squarely.		
Running scared	Behaving in ways you think will protect you from disappointments that have not yet happened (and may never happen!).		
Replaying	Rerunning and reviewing upsetting or frightening memories again and again to keep yourself on guard against being vulnerable to your mate.		

Fights that rely on manipulation tactics are a sign of stress. But, as with all stress, trying to deal with the *symptoms* alone has at best only short-term benefits. Dealing with the underlying dynamics of the relationship will have long-term consequences, since these dynamics can either aggravate or ease relationship stress. Let's look at some of them.

DYNAMICS THAT AGGRAVATE RELATIONSHIP STRESS

Projection

A man who flies into a rage if his partner procrastinates on a commitment may be fighting his own embarrassing tendency to procrastinate at the office. A woman who panics or sulks at the least sign of her mate flirting may secretly feel that she herself could take a flirtation too far. In such ways, partners may "project" their own unacceptable thoughts, feelings, and impulses onto the other. They may be hypersensitive to just those habits in their mates that they are least tolerant of in themselves.

This style of handling incidents on a daily basis can greatly increase the stress level of the relationship. Take the case of Jim.

Jim had had a bad day at the office, an annoying drive home on the crowded freeway, and an upsetting conversation with his accountant. When he finally reached home his regular parking space was occupied. Jim would feel much better if he could let off some steam, if he could find someone to blame for his day, if he could yell a bit. Jim knows, however, that this "fight" impulse is "unacceptable." In reality, there is no one to blame for his unfortunate day. He would, in fact, feel very guilty if he took out his frustrations on his wife and equally innocent children.

Solution? Perceive his *wife* as starting a fight! He searches for a look on her face that might suggest dissatisfaction or demand, and, of course, he finds it. Jim gets to have his fight and lets off steam without feeling guilty or consciously responsible. The price, however, is steep.

Displacement

By definition, displacement involves reducing potential guilt by redirecting a feeling from its original source toward a safer person or object. Have you ever kicked your cat after talking to your mother? Slammed the door while your baby was crying? Honked at innocent motorists as you mentally replayed your most recent romantic squabble? That's displacement.

Taken further, displacement can put stress on relationships. "You always hurt the one you love" can be more accurately stated as, "You only dare to hurt the one who loves you." A man who appears mild-mannered to the outside world may be touchy and quick-tempered with his mate. A woman who rages at her partner when he asks her to do something she considers excessive may not be able to raise her voice to her boss when he makes unreasonable demands on her.

Dependency

Although dependency can be healthy and a strong bond between two people, it can also be destructive and undermining. Confusing a mate with a mother or father encourages childlike reactions and muddles the present with past memories. Remember, to avoid falling into a dependent relationship that leaves one partner a child, both people must understand that there are no second chances at childhood. You can't make your mate into the parent you didn't have. Caring is, of course, different from care-taking. The former is a form of loving; the latter is manipulative and can be destructive.

Aggression

The important distinction between aggression and assertion is its intent. During assertion, we move ourselves *toward* another; during aggression, we move ourselves *against* another. Assertion is vital within a relationship. Aggression is not.

It's difficult for women to be assertive when they have been raised with the notion that they should spend their days doing office or house work, but act like the weaker sex. Many of us fear displeasing others, fear abandonment, fear appearing too independent. The truth is, reports indicate that both men and women enjoy a partner who is assertive. Such a partner eliminates the need for second-guessing and mind-reading. Such a partner gives his or her mate implicit permission to be similarly assertive. Aggression, however, often evokes more aggression—thrusts, parries, and strategies for defense.

Passivity

Passivity and evasion are not simply nonactivities that have no results. Rather, they are very manipulative and are used to seize power within the relationship without assuming the responsibility for it.

Passivity can be an aggressive act. A familiar example is the man or woman who, with an outward show of cooperation, does not accompany his or her mate to a party ("You go ahead, dear, I'll be perfectly fine here at home"), or who goes but sits passive and uninvolved. Either way, the couple is deprived of having a good time *together*.

Sexual Withdrawal

Sexual withdrawal can be seemingly passive, yet powerfully manipulative. Although most sexual dysfunctions are related to anxiety or guilt, avoiding sexual intimacy can also be an expression of disapproval or anger. Through sexual withdrawal a partner can be saying "I will not give to you, nor will I put my pleasure in your hands. I no longer feel comfortable letting you know that you can have an effect on me."

There are many problems with this dynamic. First, it sets up a pattern of bringing nonsexual problems into the bedroom. Second, it is indirect and does not effectively address the real cause of the anger. Third, it deprives *both* members of the couple, not just the partner being punished!

Sexual problems are so common among women under stress that it would be unrealistic to attribute them all to relationship stress. Some of them must be attributed to the Female Stress Syndrome as well.

SEX AND FEMALE STRESS

In his book *This Was Sex*, Sandy Teller quotes an eminent physician at the University of Pennsylvania.

> Undoubtedly man has a much more intense sexual appetite than woman. . . . With a woman, it is quite otherwise. If she is normally developed mentally, and well bred, her sexual desire is small. If this were not so, the whole world would become a brothel and marriage and family impossible.
>
> It is certain that the man that avoids women and the woman that seeks men are abnormal. Woman is wooed for her favor. She remains passive. This lies in her sexual organization and is not founded merely on dictates of good breeding.
>
> Joseph Richardson, M.D.
(and seventeen other authorities)

Although this statement was made in the year 1909, American women are *still* often expected to be sexy but not sexual, enticing but not forward, and available but not eager. American humor paints the picture vividly.

> "What does the French woman say when she is made love to?"
>
> "Oooo, la, la!"
>
> "What does the Italian woman say when she is made love to?"
>
> "Mama mia!"
>
> "What does the American woman say when she is made love to?"
>
> "Frank, the ceiling needs painting!"

Is this stereotype true? Not usually. Women share with men the capacity for sexual fantasy, desire, arousal, and satisfaction. Female orgasms involve contractions of the pubococcygeus muscles every 0.8 seconds, just as male orgasms do. In fact, women seem to have little or no refractory (unresponsive) period after orgasm, have greater sexual stamina, and are more likely to experience multiple orgasms.

Why, then, is the American woman presumed to suffer more from headaches than from desire? One reason may be male defensiveness. That is, if a man can believe that women have a low sexual drive, his own performance anxiety may be relieved. "She doesn't enjoy it anyway," he can think. "She's just going along with sex for my sake," he may want to believe.

Patricia Schreiner-Engel, assistant director of the Human Sexuality Program at Mount Sinai Medical College in New York City, points to another possible problem, which is that women, unlike men, do not have external signs of arousal to distract them from preoccupations and worries. Men see their own erections, label themselves aroused, and turn their attention to sexual pleasure. Women, however, are frequently unaware of their vaginal lubrication or genital swelling. In fact, both clinically and in her research, Schreiner-Engel finds that women often do not know how physically aroused they actually are!

Low sexual desire can be a female stress symptom for various reasons. Sometimes the stress is created by gradual life changes that have crept up over long periods of time. Sometimes the stress is related to unresolved anger and resentment toward a partner or toward men in general. Sometimes the stress is a crisis situation. Most often, chronic low sexual desire results from fears and anxieties left over from past learning.

Women in this culture seem to have been raised amid conflicting sexual messages. They face at least four different sexual dilemmas.

1. *The fear of saying "yes" vs. the fear of saying "no."* To say "yes" involves taking responsibility for birth control, monitoring male methods of contraception, or risking an unwanted pregnancy. To say "no" involves risks ranging from rape to angry rejection.

2. *Performance anxiety vs. castration concerns.* If a woman absorbs advice from her mother and the media on "How to Please Your Man," she may become a spectator during her own sexual encounters and suffer from performance anxiety severe enough to inhibit her own sexual response. If, on the other hand, she absorbs advice on "How to Maximize Your Sexual Pleasure," she runs the risk of frightening off men who may see requests as instructions, advances as aggression, interest as promiscuity, playfulness as manipulation, and passion as competition.

3. *Fear of discovery vs. fear of frustration.* Young women, older women, married women, religious women, daughters, mothers, and grandmothers all seem to be potentially embarrassed by their sexuality. There is someone, in almost every case, from whom they would prefer to hide their sexuality. More frequently than not, even hus-

bands are unaware of their wive's capacity to masturbate or fantasize. Frustration, however, is an unsatisfactory alternative, particularly since current research assures us that women, like men, have sexual needs. To deny or hide these needs may not only add to the Female Stress Syndrome, but deprive women of a natural stress antidote—satisfying sex!

4. *Dyadic duet vs. do-your-own-thing.* Humans seem to be a bonding species, and women, particularly, find themselves looking for long-term partners. Too much emphasis on finding a husband and defining oneself in terms of *his* success, however, has led to a reaction among women against the "Cinderella complex." Too much emphasis on going it alone seems to be equally unsatisfying, however. Betty Friedan suggests in her book *The Second Stage* that the trick will be to find new ways of working *with* men to build and rebuild lives, rather than bailing out of bonding altogether. Finding a balance, then, is an ongoing problem. And ongoing problems contribute to female stress and low sexual desire.

Sometimes female sexuality becomes a victim of motherhood's stresses:

    less time
    less privacy
    more distractions
    fear of another pregnancy
    self-consciousness about body changes
    concerns about adequacy as a mother

To make matters worse, a mother's own sexual desire can become a victim too. She may feel that she no longer *should* be either sexy to her husband, or sexual in her own interests. Too often, her husband may feel the same way. He would feel guilty if he allowed himself to have sexual feelings about a "mother," so he experiences a mysterious loss of desire or arousal instead—the Madonna Complex.

As sex fades from a couple's life, stress grows. An important expression of adult affection has been lost. An important source of physical pleasure has been lost. An important type of stimulation and punctuation of a routinized life has been lost. An important aspect of love has been lost. Such a couple must rediscover each other as *people*, remind themselves that they are entitled to sexual pleasure—entitled to each other!

RELATIONSHIP-STRESS MANAGEMENT

Here are some ideas for managing the stresses inherent in relationships. Some are new, some recapitulate what we have been talking about up until now. What they share is an emphasis on *realistic* expectations to help reduce chronic frustration or disappointment—realistic expectations for yourself, your mate, and your interactions.

1.   Remind your mate and yourself that you are a team—both on the same side, that of the couple!
2.   Communicate to be heard, not to win.
3.   Realize that it is not your job to teach your

mate right and wrong; teach your children, if you have them.

4. Don't confuse compliance with caring, nor lack of compliance with lack of caring.

5. Principles are rarely more important than people. Most women can find room for both!

6. Make requests, not demands. Requests are flattering and usually fulfilled. Demands are challenging, and often resisted.

7. *Ask* for what you need. Don't wait for your partner to develop mental telepathy! In the meantime, work on communication and speaking your mind. This will give your mate implicit permission to do the same, and no one will be forced to play twenty questions.

8. Develop imaginary role-reversal skills. They add empathy and sympathy to relationships. Put yourself in his place and help him understand how you see things. You will be less likely to take his behavior personally if you do.

9. Acknowledge that perfect fits do not exist; go for compromise and points for effort.

10. Recognize jealousy; it is a common human reaction. Can a father be jealous of his own children? Can a mother be jealous of her own husband? Of course. Don't deny these feelings or they will operate autonomously—treat them as real and you can give them perspective and limits.

11. Try to be self-centering. View yourself through your own eyes. Give yourself permission to relax, speak for yourself, and be good to yourself. Know yourself as you *are*, not as you think you should be. Do as Rita did:

Rita came to therapy with a list of her husband's complaints about her. She wanted help with her efforts to diet, since Don preferred her slim. She wanted help with her efforts to stop smoking, since Don couldn't tolerate cigarette butts. She wanted help becoming more organized, since Don prized efficiency. She wanted help reducing her enormous anxiety when she expected guests, since Don wanted to entertain more.

Rita had given Don the power to make her dissatisfied with most aspects of her marital functioning. Her view was off-center; it was outside-in. She was seeing herself only through his eyes.

Rita left therapy with information about how *she* felt about her weight, smoking, level of organization, and hostessing. She decided to give up smoking for her *own* sake, lose some weight as a "gift" for her husband, learn to live with the differences between her style of organization and her husband's, and to entertain whenever her husband wanted to—but by inviting guests out to a restaurant for dinner. She was pleased to be more self-accepting and surprised that Don was more accepting of her as well!

12. Try to be your own parent. It's a chance to raise yourself the way you would have wanted to be raised. Don't look to your mate to compensate for your parents' inadequacies; and don't try to parent him.

13. Permit yourself the vulnerability that comes with normal bonding. Know that you can put yourself in your partner's hands, both literally and figuratively. We bond to produce friendships. We bond to produce families. We bond to produce love.

Sometimes, no matter how much effort you put into trying to understand the dynamics of a relationship, you will not be able to alter behaviors and expectations that are firmly entrenched or operating on automatic pilot. If the problem seems to be unyielding, remember that you can always turn to professional counseling, either for yourself alone or for the two of you as a couple. A marriage counselor, sex therapist, of psychotherapist may be just what you need to help you pinpoint the sources of stress and heal a troubled relationship.

6

Mothering and the Female Stress Syndrome

Imagine this: A fourteen-hour work day. A seven-day work week. No minimum wage, no pension plan, no expense account, no promotion, no lunch hour, no drinks after work, and no paid vacation guaranteed. Men need not apply.

Sound familiar? Despite its appalling job description, American women sign up for motherhood at the rate of about 347,000 per year. It is the fringe benefits they are after: participation in creation, touching life and lives, loving, sharing, and caring. For these pay-offs they think they are willing to pay the price. Too often, however, the price is steeper in stress than they bargained for.

MOTHERING IN THE '80s

The Female Stress Syndrome is probably as old as motherhood itself. What is new is the size of the problem. Rates of both depression and anxiety reactions have been climbing among urban, suburban, and rural-dwelling homemakers since the 1940s. Furthermore, record numbers of women are choosing to postpone motherhood, forgo motherhood, or pursue a full-time career during motherhood, an option that carries its own brand of stress. Why?

Sagging Support System

Although kitchen technology has freed the homemaker from hours of physical labor, progress has created problems too. Harriet's experiences are common.

> Harriet left the small Ohio town where she had grown up to attend Boston University in Massachusetts. Through her new roommate, she was introduced to Alex, a New Yorker attending Harvard Business School. They dated through his remaining two years at Harvard and then married. Alex became an account executive for a national corporation and was asked to locate in Atlanta, Georgia. Within thirty-two months of leaving her home, Harriet had moved, married, moved again, and suspended her education, and was now pregnant. She did part-time work during her pregnancy in order to save a little extra money for baby costs and found little time to meet her new neighbors or continue her education. By the time the baby arrived, Harriet was feeling alone and stressed.

Separated from her extended family and hometown, Harriet was separated from an important mothering support system. Years ago, motherhood was shared by many generations, and a new mother was helped by her own mother and even her grandmother. Now, however, families are usually split into units small enough to move to locations that offer jobs.

Instead of turning to her mother and grandmother for advice, today's mobile young homemaker must turn to the "experts." Unfortunately, when she does, she gets too much information. "How to" books are everywhere. Child experts speak from car radios, television sets, and cassette tapes and write newspaper columns and magazine features.

The mass media have replaced grandmother! But whereas grandmother's advice was consistent, today's myriad experts offer myriad opinions. The young mother is soon completely confused, lacking the traditional support system.

The Working Mother

Fifty-one percent of the women in this country, many of them mothers, held jobs as of 1979. Some were married, and some were divorced, single, or widowed. Most were working, because the American dream of "getting somewhere" had been replaced by the reality of working hard to avoid falling behind.

Working may help women relieve the family budget squeeze, but it also contributes to stress. Women do not trade in housework for job work; they *add* job duties to home and mothering duties.

Working mothers often worry that they may be cheating their families of their time, and so they try to make it up to them. This in turn leaves the working mother even more tired, still guilt-ridden, and without any time for herself.

Often working mothers must deal also with sexism—and not just sexism at their place of employment, either. Many women report that as working mothers they are discriminated against by their children's teachers, school committee members, and neighbors, and within their own families by critical parents, in-laws, or even husbands.

Betti-Anne and Joe had four children. They both agreed that the children needed Betti-Anne at home full time, but as Joe's salary increments fell behind cost-of-living increases, Betti-Anne had to take a nine-to-five job. Soon after starting work, Betti-Anne was called to school by the teacher of her oldest son. The teacher reported that the boy seemed to be having difficulty concentrating on his classwork. She suggested that Betti-Anne's new job and schedule might be upsetting her son and interfering with his ability to concentrate.

Feeling upset and guilty, Betti-Anne called the boy's grandparents and received two versions of what she calls the "Mother's Place Is in the Home" lecture. Her husband suggested that they increase discipline and not indulge the boy. Betti-Anne's best friend disagreed and suggested family counseling.

Things did not improve until a state-wide intelligence test given in school showed that Betti-Anne's son was extremely gifted and probably very bored in the classroom. His classroom problems co-incided with his mother's new job, but were not caused by her working. He was skipped a grade, Betti-Anne kept her job, and all was well. Or was it? Betti-Anne learned how quickly her working could be held responsible for her family's problems. She also learned how ready she was to do the same. Would she feel less guilty the next time a problem came up?

The alternative seems to create stress as well. That is, a mother who chooses to stay home runs the risk of feeling that she is not doing her share to relieve her husband of the economic strain of these times. Furthermore, her sense of dependency is heightened even as she clips coupons, buys on sale, and pinches pennies. It seems that mothers in the '80s are likely to feel stressed and guilty if they do work outside the house, and stressed and guilty if they do not.

Divorced, single, and widowed mothers, of course, usually have very little choice about whether they work. The cost of raising a child from birth to about eighteen years on a moderate budget has been estimated to be at least $50,000, excluding childbirth and college costs; and since the cost of a well-educated mother not working during those same years is *at least* $75,000 in lost income, it is obvious that money stress is considerable in single-parent households.

A different kind of stress is created for modern mothers by what I'll call "Dana's Dilemma." Dana is a friend who confided recently, "I'd be much happier at home than I am working." Since financial considerations were not the motivation for Dana's job, I asked why she did not remain at home. "I feel that being a wife and a mother is my thing, but I don't have any friends to do my thing *with* anymore," she replied.

It seems that most of Dana's friends left the PTA

and the A&P in order to return to school or pursue careers. In fact, they scolded Dana for not doing the same. Social pressure on women to "do their own thing," Dana claims, apparently does not encompass staying home and mothering!

"A Mother's Work Is Never Done . . ."

Current popular social pressures on women to reject the conventional sex-roles often mean that mothers and homemakers feel the stress of low status. Since women need no experience, no entrance exam, no prerequisites, no courses, and no degrees to become mothers, the role is frequently thought to be low in prestige and exclusiveness—and not just by men (see "Dana's Dilemma," page 106). Compare our culture to New Guinea, for example, where Margaret Mead found that men so envy and value motherhood that they hold ceremonies in which they pretend to give birth! Similarly, the Kung nomads of the Kalahari Desert have considered child care as a joint male and female activity for more than a thousand years.

Here in the Western world, however, we see things differently. Furthermore, the average homemaker spends between fifty and seventy-five hours a week on housecleaning and other physical labor: bending, pulling, pushing, zipping, wiping, catching, patching, lifting, lugging, and hugging. Since when has physical labor added to the attractiveness of a social position?

It is true that women no longer have to bake their own bread or churn ice cream for the kiddies, but just look at the list of chores that still must be done.

HOUSEHOLD TASKS
(after R. Stafford, E. Backman, and P. Dibona)

cooking
dusting
dishwashing
vacuuming
laundering
scrubbing floors,
   windows, etc.
bathing children
managing finances
feeding children
shopping, menu
   planning
repairing or arranging
   repairs

lawn tending
feeding spouse
picking up after the
   family
disciplining
organizing children's
   play
arranging for baby-
   sitters
managing garbage and
   trash
snow removal
feeding pets

Beyond Housework

Beyond household duties are the stresses that include loss of freedom, some isolation, and much monotony. Not that these problems are exclusive to the mother—the secretary, executive, and cab driver may have the same complaints. An important difference, though, is that the secretary, executive, and cab driver have other adults around; the full-time mother usually does not. She waits all day for her husband, who may be too tired to talk when he returns home from work.

The list of stresses associated with mothering goes on and on. Listen to the mothers who meet with me weekly to discuss stress management.

"I feel like I am always 'on duty.'"
"I am always trying to be the *perfect* mother!"

"I worry about accidents all the time. If the children are late, I think the worst."

"When I am on vacation, I don't miss my children. Is this normal? It makes me feel guilty."

"Saying no is hardest—even when I know that I am right."

"Coordinating everyone's time schedules drives me crazy."

"I resent the fact that I'm running the family, but am letting the children think that Daddy is in charge!"

"Having to have answers for my children wears me out."

"I hate being responsible for discipline every day. I'm always the bad guy."

"If my children don't stop fighting with each other soon, I'm leaving home!"

"I don't mind the housework—it's balancing the checkbook I hate."

"I'm always afraid someone will ask me what I 'do for a living' at a party; I'll have to say 'nothing' when I really do *everything*!"

"My husband thinks relaxing means watching television at night. Where does that leave me?"

"I don't think I exist for the world. All the mail is for my husband!"

MOTHER'S STRESS CHECKLIST

Nine-to-five hours? Call in for a sick day? Maternity leave from maternity? Not a chance! High risk for the Female Stress Syndrome? Without a doubt!

If you are a mother, fill out this mother's stress

checklist and see how high a risk you're running. To the left of each item, write your points according to the following scale:

---

0 NEVER TRUE
1 RARELY TRUE
2 SOMETIMES TRUE
3 FREQUENTLY TRUE
4 ALWAYS TRUE

ACTIVITIES

———— I can completely lose interest in social activities and hobbies; the effort seems too great.

———— I find it difficult to know what I would like to do with free time.

———— I forget what chore I have started and don't follow through with plans.

———— I start more projects than I can possibly finish.

———— I feel the house must be spotless and run with complete efficiency.

———— I find myself feeling overwhelmed and out of control because there are too many demands on me.

———— I find it hard to say no to my children or husband, even when I think I am right to say no.

SELF-CONCEPT

———— I feel that my appearance doesn't really matter to me or anyone else.

——— I feel that there is very little time for me in my day.

——— I think other people's opinions are more valid than mine.

——— I feel unappreciated by my family.

——— I fantasize about what my life would be like if I could start again.

——— I find I exaggerate and boast to friends.

——— I feel a sense of resentment and anger that I cannot really explain.

——— I find that I often look for compliments and praise.

APPETITE

——— I feel too aggravated or tense to eat.

——— I crave coffee or cigarettes to keep me going.

——— I binge and then regret it.

——— I need chocolate and/or other carbohydrates when I feel tired or down.

——— I suffer from nausea, cramps, or diarrhea.

——— I snack too often.

SLEEP

——— I have trouble falling asleep.

——— I awaken earlier than I need/want to.

——— I have nightmares.

——— I do not feel rested even when I have a full night's sleep.

——— I fall asleep earlier than I want to in the evening.

111

——— I seem to need a nap in the afternoon.
——— I awaken during the night.

OUTLOOK

——— I feel like I've lost my sense of humor.
——— I feel impatient and irritable.
——— I cry without knowing why.
——— I relive the past.
——— I am pessimistic about the future.
——— I feel numb and emotionless.
——— I find myself laughing nervously, too loudly, or without reason.
——— I ignore things that would upset me.
——— I am sorry that I chose motherhood.

——— TOTAL

If your score is between *1 and 40*, congratulations! You are at *low risk* for the Female Stress Syndrome, since you seem to have a sense of control and are managing your maternal career well.

If your score is between *41 and 75*, you are probably *mildly stressed* by mothering and may experience some transient stress symptoms.

If your score is between *76 and 110*, you are running a *moderate risk* for the Female Stress Syndrome. Use the self-help advice in this book to lower your stress levels.

If your score is between *111 and 148*, you are in the *high stress* range, and this book is particularly important for you!

MANAGING MOTHERHOOD

What to do when a mother is burned-out blue? What to do when she feels taken for granted, tired, unappreciated, and unattractive? What to do if that mother is you?

Begin by reexamining your role honestly. List the advantages of motherhood for *you*. Perhaps it is nurturing, perhaps feeling needed, perhaps being in control, perhaps being an authority figure, perhaps shaping decisions, perhaps being in the center of a family, or perhaps enjoying children's activities yourself. As your sense of choice about motherhood increases, stress stimulated by resentment will decrease.

Then reexamine your expectations for yourself as a mother. Are you realistic? How closely do your priorities match your routines? Which of these elements needs adjusting? (Often this is not an easy question to answer, so give it a lot of thought.)

In addition, every mother must become her own sympathetic permission-giver. Do you usually feel that you must be overworked and overtired before you let yourself rest? Do you feel that you have to justify time off to your husband, your mother-in-law, and the rest of the world? Was your hospital stay after the birth of your last child your last morning in bed? *Why?*

Mothers who wait to be rescued by others become disappointed, angry, and stressed: disappointed because any rescue that does come will probably not be well timed; angry because they have given a great deal of power to others; stressed because they must continually show the world that they need rescuing. Mothers who feel entitled to rest, relaxation, and realistic expectations can give themselves the permission they need to avoid the Female Stress Syndrome. They can be good to themselves. They can appreciate attention and considerateness from others as important extras, rather than as too little, too late.

7

Stress and the Working Woman

THE NEW WOMAN

It was estimated at the beginning of this decade that approximately 90 percent of the female population has worked or will work for pay at some time in their lives. Does this statistic surprise you? A number of interesting factors combine to make the percentage so high.

Birth Control

For the first time in history, women control the timing of their children. The time before, in between, and after childbirth and child raising can be planned to a greater extent than ever before.

Kitchen Technology

Modern materials and machines save time, energy, and physical wear and tear. Convenience foods reduce cooking time—or even eliminate it altogether.

Reexamination of Anatomical Destiny

It has occurred to many people that if a woman can work and bring home a paycheck, a man can manage a household and raise children. Since we are living in a postindustrial society, most jobs today are service jobs that require brains rather than brawn. Even in physical work, such as firefighting or military combat training, women are proving their ability to hold their own. By choice or by necessity, both sexes are broadening their views about what different people can do for a living.

Inflation and Recession

Two incomes are not only better than one—they will probably be necessary to maintain a decent standard of living in the future and to carry a family over a period of strikes or unemployment.

Divorce

As you are undoubtedly aware by now, the divorce rate stands at 50 percent. No more can women count on "lifetime employment" as housewives or homemakers; nor, on the other hand, can they count on alimony. Alimony is going out of style—legally, practically, and socially. Divorced women work to support themselves, their children, and, often, their independence. Working provides the financial base for life choices that are alternatives to remarriage.

"Dutch Treat" Marriages

Women are staying single longer now than ever before. Their finances develop with their careers, and they see themselves as self-supporting individuals. The women's movement, of course, has reinforced the idea of personal autonomy in the economic as well as the emotional sphere—for both sexes. Thus, when one of these women ties the knot, the result is often what I call a "dutch treat" marriage. Both husband and wife maintain their own finances as when they were single, or they share expenses according to convenience or individual income.

For all these twentieth-century developments, however, the high percentage of working women really represents a *reentry* of women into the job market, not a new entry. Think about your own roots. You will most likely remember that your grandmothers and great-grandmothers worked. They may have managed the family business, worked in a shop, farmed, done domestic or factory work. In fact, the postwar '50s and '60s was probably one of the few periods in history when most women didn't have to work, since the economic boom during that era meant that one income was sufficient to support a whole family. The catch phrase "New Woman," then, could better be rephrased as "Renewed Woman."

NINE-TO-FIVE PLUS

Although women have reentered the job market, research backs up women's own observations that they are still expected to execute their traditional roles at home as well as their duties at work. M. J. Luetgert found in a survey of five hundred men and women that the majority of his sampling advocated greater career involvement for women *and* retention of domestic duties. And don't think professional marriages are any different. In 1976, R. B. Bryson and associates reported in the *American Psychologist* that husbands who were doctors and lawyers were no more helpful to their wives who worked than were nonprofessional husbands.

Working women carry out dual roles in response to their own expectations, as well as their husbands' expectations. We have learned our roles through custom and culture, through models and reinforcement, and we are no less hard on ourselves than are those around us. We run from board meetings to PTA meetings, monitor ticker tape and supermarket receipts, deal with demanding supervisors and recalcitrant repair people, and rarely question our dual responsibilities. We are stressed and resentful, driven and guilt-ridden, and we are convinced that that's the way things are supposed to be.

DUAL ROLES, DUAL STRESSES

Working women with dual roles are stressed in ways not usually shared by working men, or by nonworking women.

For one thing, although grandmothers and great-grandmothers may have worked, many mothers in the '50s did not. Therefore there are few role models for today's working mothers. If they *were* employed, women were expected to hold jobs, not develop careers! Career development takes long-range planning and commitment. It can mean sacrificing immediate benefits, such as a high-paying but dead-end job, for long-term gain. It can mean playing the politics of the office. It means competing with others—and the others are generally men.

Furthermore, in past generations women were expected to be seen and not heard at the office. Their traditional jobs are secretaries, receptionists, typists, and clerks placed them in helpful, supportive, servicing roles. It is no surprise, then, that as women have entered competitive, career-track jobs, they have met with resistance and resentment in the work place.

Although being a full-time homemaker has its own stresses, in some ways it is the easier side of the coin. Compare the role of wife or parent to that of a working woman. As a wife or parent

- No exams, prerequisites, or previous experience are necessary.
- There is no need to submit a resume for the job.
- Failures are usually not observed, analyzed, and judged in public. They can be hidden in the privacy of the home.
- There is no competition on the job. The laundry is all yours!
- There is no competition *for* the job. Your children are all yours!
- There is no time clock. Your schedule is yours to

structure—no doubt it's filled beyond the waking hours, but it is still all yours.

- You are your own supervisor and boss. This is not to say that you are not your severest critic and slave-driver. On the contrary, at home you probably assume more responsibility than if you did have a boss. It is a different kind of stress trade-off, however, than that involved in working under a boss.

Working women who are wives and/or mothers often live with a sharp conflict between their roles inside and outside the home. Many mothers who work part time report that they cannot feel satisfied in either role. When they are working, they can think only of the child at home. When they are home, they feel they should be on the job.

Women who work full time, on the other hand, may feel guilty that they were away from home all day. When they come home, they begin to compensate rather than relax. They put in extra effort and activity at home as if they had been playing all day.

Of course, arriving home after a hard day at the office, women can feel resentful of children's and husbands' demands—and then feel distressed by their own resentment! Too often this leads to an ongoing marital debate about whose job or income is more important to the family's survival. Since the husband's income is usually designated for the utilities and other running costs, and the wife's income more often provides the "extras," husbands seem to have the upper hand. If the discrepancy in income is sizable, the debate may have some minor merit. If there is little discrepancy in income, however, the two paychecks might just as well be considered part of a pool of financial resources. The "extras" that a wife's income provides, moreover, usually turn out to be such nonfrivolous items as the family car, the family trip, and even the family's food. Jenny's case is not uncommon.

> Jenny's husband took paternalistic pride in her early successes as a dress designer. He helped her make contacts and develop bookkeeping skills. As her business grew, he was less needed and she was less available. She had her own stories to tell and her own business trips to take. He demanded that she choose between her business and him. She offered him the same choice to point out the absurdity of his request. He, of course, said he could never give up his business and that his involvement in it did not mean that he did not love her. She said the same was true for her. "It's different for a woman," he replied. "I'm sorry to hear that you feel that way," she said. She also said goodbye.

Not all women would, could, or should say goodbye in a situation like Jenny's. Not all women would find themselves in such a situation. Too many, however, do. Too many must then struggle with realistic alternatives. My most heartfelt professional advice to such women is this: If you are thinking of leaving your marriage because you would prefer to live *alone* than to live with the stress of the relationship, a separation may work for you. If, however, you are leaving your marriage for a fantasy of another, more perfect husband—reconsider. People are package deals, and we cannot order the options to suit us at will. Job and marriage coordination creates problems for all of us; don't jump to blame the stress on your spouse.

Even in an ideal relationship, coordinating job and marriage can be difficult.

Ruth trains employees for a cosmetics firm and loves her job. Jim is chagrined, however, that his wife is not being paid what she is worth. "She should quit and go where she is appreciated," he insists. "They think she will work for next to nothing because they know that her work is not a financial necessity." "Please don't pressure me, Jim," Ruth repeats constantly. "More money will mean I'll have to take my work more seriously. I'm pretending it's a wonderful game right now. I don't feel guilty if I leave early to go shopping with my kids. More money will mean more anxiety. You earn enough for both of us." "That's not the point," Jim replies.

And Jim is right. Ruth's pay should reflect her worth, not her needs. Her ambivalence stems from her job-marriage conflicts, not her economic philosophy. What does her low pay indicate about her boss's view of female employees? Would it be different if Ruth were, indeed, "in need"? Probably not!

NOT JUST ONE OF THE GUYS

Whether a woman is married or not, childless or not, the nature of the on-the-job stress is part of what separates the "girls" from the "guys." The sources of this stress are many, but the most prevalent are the fear of success and the problem of sexism.

The handicapping effect of the fear of success has been widely analyzed. *It is real.* Given society's emphasis on appearance and passivity in females, working women may fear that career or job success will make them less attractive. Unfortunately, research bears them out. Even more unfortunately, this stereotyping is practiced by women as well as men. It's not uncommon to find people automatically labeling feminists as "ugly." In reality, feminists are not self-selected for looks—they cover the full range of possible appearances. And in one study (N. Costrich, J. Feinstein, and L. Kidder, 1975), written character sketches were evaluated by both male and female subjects: assertive women were judged as less likable than passive women by both sexes.

The origins of women's fear of success, then, are not mysterious. Many were discussed in Chapter 4, "Nonassertiveness Training and the Female Stress Syndrome." Others are personal to each individual. Sexism, however, is universal and affects us all in the same ways.

Sexism comes in many forms, some subtle, some overt.

- Demeaning comments depicting women as sex objects.
- Vulgar jokes meant to embarrass women and place them in a position of being a spoilsport if they object, and feeling humiliated if they don't.
- Condescension by men, whatever their relative position or rank in the office; intimidation by tone.
- Misuse of "occupational power" by men who will make sexual innuendos and advances toward women who lack job security or union protection.
- Job discrimination, precipitating two types of

stress: the stress of gathering evidence and seeking legal redress, and the stress of deciding whether or not to pursue that course.

• Expressions of domination-aggression, which can lower our sense of worth unless addressed.

As Linda was given more executive power in her media job, her second-in-command more frequently rolled up the morning newspaper and "playfully" tapped her behind with it as she passed his desk. "Just kidding," he would say when she expressed annoyance. "You're too sensitive, Linda." She finally returned the gesture as he entered a board meeting. "Just kidding," she sweetly intoned. You can guess the rest.

There is a direct link between sexism and female stress. As our sense of control is lowered, our sense of stress is increased, and the very focus of sexism is the lowering of women's control over their own lives. We feel that we have little power to influence our occupational destiny. Exposure to sexism fosters stress, and fighting sexism increases it. It's a real "catch-22" situation.

THE TYPE A WOMAN

Given the special stresses that working, career, and professional women are subject to, it is no wonder that they experience female stress symptoms. Given the special drive and character women must have to compete successfully and even to excel in the working world, it is no wonder that they suffer "executive stress" symptoms as well.

According to Meyer Friedman and Ray Rosenman, achievement-oriented male executives have long paid for their personality profile with high blood pressure and/or heart disease. The same characteristics that were reinforced by their career successes were making them susceptible to psychosomatic diseases. These characteristics include

competitiveness
aggressiveness
secret anger
impatience and
    irritability
perfectionism

constant raising of their
    own quotas
focus on approval of
    others for their self-
    esteem

Friedman and Rosenman labeled this profile the Type A personality, and warned Type A men of their high risk for stress-related symptoms.

Now, as women are entering executive careers, they are exhibiting their own brand of Type A behavior. Imagine the Type A personality as a working woman, and the result is the following:

- She is a perfectionist, and so must be the perfect employee without slacking off as beauty, devoted daughter, lover, wife, mother, friend.
- She is never satisfied with her achievements.
- She is as impatient and irritable as the Type A man, but unfortunately has less time and more chores to be impatient and irritable about!
- She can be aggressive rather than assertive.
- She gives others enormous power to affect her feelings about herself through their reactions to her.

- She is secretly angry that no man is saving her from herself, although she would like to feel differently.
- She competes on the job as well as with other mothers and wives.
- She schedules a dinner party for the day after her quarterly presentation to the board, since all her roles are priority roles.

When a man exhibits Type A behavior, physicians and family become concerned. "Get a thorough checkup," they say. "Take two weeks' vacation." However, this advice is not as readily applied to Type A women, most of whom have family and social responsibilities they can't easily escape—or which they *feel* they can't easily escape, which amounts to the same thing. Too often, they simply find themselves settling for the notion that everything will look a lot better after a good night's sleep.

A good night's sleep can't hurt, but it will not be enough to reduce the stress symptoms of a Type A woman. Better advice? First of all, educate yourself. Educate yourself about stress in general; about your particular stress pattern; about the opportunities for stress management in your daily life. Take *control* of your life, in fact and in spirit. Don't give others the power to affect your self-esteem and behavior with their approval or disapproval. Decide for yourself how you feel about yourself. Don't give others the power to control your time schedule unless it is appropriate. Don't give others the power to control your goals through implicit or explicit competition. You must concentrate on winning your own self-approval, scheduling your time yourself, and setting and achieving your own goals.

Try to make the switch from evaluating and judging yourself to describing and accepting yourself. The former increases stress, the latter gives you a chance to manage it. You might not be able to change your Type A behavior easily, but you can at least allow for it, work around it, and recognize it. You can catch yourself in the middle of becoming a spectator of your own performance. You can smile at your own Cinderella fantasies. You can switch your assertiveness from off-putting demands to flattering requests. But you can do these things only if you know yourself. If you are caught up in a flood of self-evaluation and self-criticism instead, you'll be too busy steering to chart your own course and feel in control of your own destination.

On the very practical side, here are some suggestions from other working women.

1. Buy more clothes and underwear to avoid the need for frequent laundry and cleaning trips. Include dark soil-resistant suits and lots of extra blouses. Give yourself permission to stock up! You save time for every penny you spend.
2. Hire help, as much as you can afford. Find a cleaning service. Let the tailor fix your hems, the laundry do your shirts. Have a fashion consultant identify a few types of clothing that always look good on you to simplify your shopping. Or use a professional shopper if your department offers this service. Use caterers or waiters and bartenders for parties.

Teenagers and college students are good sources for many of these services. Don't overlook a tax accountant and a travel agent. In the long run, these services are cheaper than the doctor's bills that may follow too much stress.

3. Schedule escape. Read a novel in the bath, on the bus, or at lunchtime. If your body can't go to a faraway island, at least your psyche can!

4. Find private time. One half hour after everyone else has gone to sleep or before everyone else has awakened can be *your* time for indulgence, contemplation, or fun.

5. Play. If you enjoy games, take a crossword puzzle to breakfast, or backgammon to dinner. Psychologist Constance Freeman and her associates have relaxed during ongoing lunchtime Scrabble games for eight years!

6. If you have a mate who works, establish a policy of "equal flexibility." Each of you must be able to take it for granted that your goal is to share the total load of household work equally, and that both your schedules and energy levels may vary unpredictably. For example, once you have this understanding, whoever had the easier day or who got home first would prepare the dinner. If neither of you has time or energy, you might go out, order in, or even eat separately.

Practicality is the key. It is important that working couples not let practical tasks such as cooking and cleaning become symbols for other things, such as loving and caring. When both partners have equally heavy schedules, let meals be for nourishment and count on conversation, sex, consideration, and the like to demonstrate your love and caring for each other.

7. Determine the healthiest diet for you and make sure you have the right foods on hand. Do you need a protein snack at 4 P.M.? Does your favorite diet call for only cottage cheese at breakfast? Again, stock up! You will be much less stress-prone if your body has the nutrients it needs, and you have the satisfaction of sticking to your diet. Make it easy for yourself.

8. Keep lists. Whether in the form of a small notebook or pocket calendar that is always in your purse, or a more elaborate categorizing technique taught by some of the time-management courses, such a system will enable you to trap thoughts, names, addresses, dates, and so on as they come to you and to get things done efficiently. Again, taking control of your environment lowers stress.

9. In an article entitled "Type A Behavior: A Progress Report," Meyer Friedman gives the following suggestion: practice walking, talking, and driving your car at a *slower pace*. This can help to reduce your sense of urgency and, consequently, reduce irritation and even anger. It may force you to schedule fewer activities and leave you more time for "joy and affection in situations that previously either irritated or angered."

10. Self-hypnosis and other special relaxation ex-

ercises can be a great help in relieving tension. See Chapter 10, page 186, for more about these.

THE BENEFITS OF WORKING

Hard as it may be to believe, despite all the stresses associated with working its benefits are enormous. An important antidote to the Female Stress Syndrome is the kind of support system most work environments offer—the network of co-workers. This support system serves many functions on many levels.

- Working can provide social contacts and a sense of belonging. Spending almost half your waking life during the week with any group of people is bound to facilitate ties. Spending it sharing goals, hard work, anxieties, and victories can make for very strong ties. Sometimes lifelong friends are made at work. Sometimes the friendships are unique to the work place. Either way, the relationships can be valuable and supportive. Either way, you are part of a team: a department, a company, an industry, or a profession. A fundamental need for belonging is to some degree filled.
- Working can provide different points of view. There is never one reality or one view of reality. Talking about problems with your work network can broaden your perspective on any topic. It can help you understand another's behavior in a less personalized way. It can help you re-interpret last night's domestic fight or this

morning's news bulletin. It can bring you into conversation with men and women from other backgrounds, generations, and businesses. It can exasperate you and fascinate you and help to make your thinking more flexible.

- Working can provide humor. Heard any good jokes lately? If so, and if you work, you probably heard them at the office. Office jokes travel by word of mouth, by phone, and even by photocopies. Cartoons are posted. Gags are pulled. Office war-stories and office histories are shared. Tense tales become comedies in the retelling, and looking at the light side is an important fringe benefit of the working life.

- Working can provide resources. Your workmates may have ideas, information, and know-how that you do not, and vice versa. Pooling resources, in fact, has become almost a ritual in many work situations involving women. Sometimes the aim is career information and opportunities; sometimes more personal needs are met. Either way, the more information and knowledge you can gather, the more control you will have. And the more control, the less stress!

- Working can provide confidants. Who understands your work frustrations and elations better than someone who is also on the job? Who would be safer to talk to about family problems than someone who is *not* in the family? In both cases, a workmate can be a valuable ally. Have you noticed that it is sometimes easier to unburden yourself to a semistranger about a personal sorrow than it is to those close to you?

- Working can provide cushioning and escape

valves for anger. This can work in two different ways. First, work can provide an opportunity to use constructively the adrenaline generated by anger. You can tear into your work, instead of into your mother-in-law. You can beat a deadline instead of a dead issue. You can argue for a proposal, instead of arguing against your husband. You can leave your desk phone instead of your boyfriend.

Second, anger that feels inappropriate at home may be entirely legitimate at the office. You may not feel it is constructive to get angry at a spouse or child for performing poorly, but you can do so constructively and systematically at the office, where grievance and evaluation procedures are formalized.

- Working can provide sympathy. The communal expressions of sympathy for sorrow that you get from the office are a unique source of support. Your workmates are a semipublic group, wider than your family yet not as impersonal as strangers or polite neighbors. The larger the group, furthermore, the more likely that you will find others who have experienced the same sorrow. You can see why retirement means far more than separation from work. It means separation from a network, as well.

- Working can provide adult conversation and intellectual stimulation. Do you spend most of your time talking with children? Do you spend most of your day hearing *Sesame Street* and Mister Rogers educating infants? Do you consider the verbal exchange at the gas station the most adult conversation of your day? Then you will understand how important this aspect of working is. Many women take part-time jobs or volunteer their work just to spend at least part of their day with other adults. For most women, who work because they must work, intellectual stimulation is not the aim, but it is always an important fringe benefit.

- Working can provide a source of praise and reassurance. Too often, good or extra work at home is taken for granted or goes unnoticed altogether. Although this is possible on the job too, more often you will be told if your work is good. Promotions and paychecks are tangible proof of performance. Even women who enjoyed being homemakers for its own sake are thrilled with their enhanced sense of worth when they return to work in their later years. They enjoy feeling that they can contribute to the family in a financial way. They enjoy the power that accompanies any position. They enjoy putting their many skills on public display.

- Working can provide objective feedback. Your own family, appreciative or otherwise, can't really be considered objective. In the work place, you and your work are evaluated often, by many people who have no interest in you other than how effectively you are doing your job. You can base further actions and decisions on impartial data, which increases your sense of identity and control. A great stress reliever!

In the past, the extended family helped to prevent stress buildup by serving all these functions. Now, in a way, we must each create our own extended "families," our networks, our support systems. Whether you work outside the home or not, think about each of the ten network functions mentioned. Are there some that you're not getting through your work, friends, or family associations? If so, actively seek people to add to your support system who can help provide what you need. The quality of your life may depend on it.

The benefits of working go far beyond networking. Entering the marketplace with your skills means negotiating a price tag for your work. For most women, an increase in salary or commission means an increase in self-esteem. A paycheck is a tangible statement of work, a source of pride and some degree of independence.

Raised in an era when girls were taught "you are who you marry," women in their forties and fifties often find that working at a career or profession helps them reaffirm their identity. Women at workshops tell me that working outside the home finally provides them with an answer to that perennial cocktail-party question, "And what do you do?" Many women choose to work as homemakers for many years, then move on to their next commitment. Many others have not yet married or have decided not to marry. For these women, work is even more primary to their identity. For still other women, work and love (with or without marriage) are equally vital. The key is to know yourself and what you want; to be aware of both the problems and the benefits inherent in your choice; and to seek to reduce the stresses in the ways suggested here, as well as in any other ways that work for you.

8

Hidden Stresses

They are all around, distracting you, wearing away at your patience, creating anxious anticipation. They produce fatigue, irritability, and tension. They are subtle, however; they sometimes hit and run. They are the hidden stresses contributing to the Female Stress Syndrome.

HIDDEN STRESS #1: DRIVING

Merle glanced at the clock and realized that she had not left enough time for the ride to her daughter's nursery school. She grabbed her coat and bag, ran to the car, and pulled out of her driveway into traffic. She noticed that she did not have time to fill up the gas tank. For the rest of the trip, one eye was on the tank indicator, and one ear was listening for a sputtering engine.

Her thoughts were on the inconvenience to her daughter's teacher created by her lateness, and she increased her speed. Within a half minute, Merle heard a siren behind her. Her heart seemed to jump as she searched the rear view mirror for a police car. Instead she saw an ambulance, and pulled over to the side of the road to permit its passage. Now she was even more late. Again Merle merged into traffic and picked up speed. Just as she did so, the car on her right crossed into her lane without signaling. Merle swerved automatically and came close to creating her own accident. She was now stuck behind this car and forced to inch along or to pass on the right illegally.

She passed, picked up speed again, and rushed to a red light. The light seemed to be the longest she had ever encountered, and she decided it was broken. She was about to risk going through the red light when it changed to green. She started up again, only to be stopped three more times by long red lights.

To avoid more lights, Merle turned off the main road onto a narrow suburban street and found within minutes that she was blocked by a garbage truck making pickups. She wanted to scream, or to cry. Either would have felt better than sitting in her car like a prisoner while her daughter and her teacher waited endlessly in the schoolyard.

Does Merle's adventure sound familiar? Short-distance driving is a major source of stress, and suburban women must deal with this stress daily. Much of their day is spent chauffeuring: to the dentist; to get the children haircuts; to the train station and back again;

to play-overs, sleep-overs, and eat-overs; to the movies; to town; to the supermarket; to the school; to the post office or the cleaners; and to the service station so that the chauffeuring will not be interrupted by car problems. (When it *is* interrupted by car problems, more stress!)

Since stress increases as control and predictability decrease, driving is one of the most stressful of daily activities. It demands high levels of visual-motor skills, good judgment, vigilance, experience, caution, technical knowledge, and a defensive mentality. The consequences associated with mistakes in this activity range from costly repair to encounters with the law to bodily harm and death.

Even if one's own driving is completely adequate, consider all the other problems that can upset control and predictability while driving:

> horn blasts from other motorists
> sirens and flashing lights from emergency or police vehicles
> unanticipated swerves and switches by another driver
> sudden blowouts or slow tire-leaks
> engine troubles
> accidents producing inconvenience, tie-ups, or danger
> unsafe road and weather conditions and unsafe roads
> school buses, which cannot be passed
> slow drivers, speeders, and tailgaters
> wrong turns, poor directions, and red lights
> male drivers

HIDDEN STRESS #2: WAITING

In a survey of more than four hundred women, "waiting" was consistently listed as a not-so-hidden pet peeve. Most women, whether they are urban or suburban, feel that many of their most frustrating minutes are spent waiting. Waiting for what? Waiting for people: their mates or their dates, their children, repairers and preparers. If they are mothers they wait for baby-sitters and pediatricians. If they are working women they wait on bank lines, elevator lines, and commuter lines. Even the ladies' room at a theater has a longer line than the men's room! Low control? Yes. High stress? Absolutely.

HIDDEN STRESS #3: ENTERTAINING

Another source of female burnout is entertaining. This is typically "women's work," and it is certainly filled with labor: shopping, cleaning, dicing, cooking, serving, setting, and cleaning (again). It is also filled with stress.

The stresses associated with entertaining vary, of course, from time to time, and from woman to woman, but a number of generalizations can be made.

1. Preparing your own food involves the risk of outcomes ranging from "nothing special" to "disaster." Thus, stress occurs because of the low predictability factor.
2. Coordinating the timing of many dishes and many guests can tax your sense of control.

3. Entertaining on short notice adds time pressures and interferes with the planning process.
4. Entertaining strangers raises additional problems. It is difficult to predict their food preferences, their humor, and their interests. If the strangers are business associates, it is difficult to predict the importance of the visit. If the strangers are new family members or new acquaintances, you may feel that you are being judged.
5. Entertaining in-laws: performance stress.
6. Entertaining friends: competition stress.
7. Entertaining children: thankless stress.
8. Entertaining during holidays: according to researcher Thomas Holmes, the most stressful of all. In fact, he considers Christmas a stressful life event. High expectations, high expenses, and high numbers of family interactions are probably to blame.

HIDDEN STRESS #4: NOISE

Men suffer from noise pollution too, of course, but women often have their own special recipe for this type of hidden stress.

Mix: An alarm clock ringing, two teenagers bickering, a husband grunting, a shower running, a baby crying.

Add: A coffee pot whistling, a telephone ringing, a school bus honking.

Blend: Pet noises, television noises, radio noises, vacuum cleaner noises, washing machine noises, clothes dryer noises.

Optional: Hair dryer drone, food processor noises, siblings screaming, car-pool and/or full-house hubbub, disposal crunches, door-slamming, toy-breaking, assorted neighborhood noises.

Some women even find that they have a special knack for listening for noise—never mind the noises that are simply thrust upon them. They always have an ear cocked for sounds of trouble from their children, for nuances of neediness from their friends, for sounds from their babies as they breathe during the night. It's not just the noise that bothers women, it's the fact that these sounds signal special responsibilities that they generally bear alone. The wear and tear of aural monitoring, despite this rather lighthearted discussion, must be taken seriously. Research leaves no doubt that noises of this nature affect concentration, irritability, and the capacity to cope.

HIDDEN STRESS #5: PHOBIAS

Phobias add a great deal of stress to many women's daily lives. A phobia is an unrealistic fear or unrecognized avoidance pattern that can complicate coping and trigger Female Stress Syndrome symptoms.

For some women, these hidden stresses are holdovers from their childhood. Ingrid describes her phobia like this.

I was in bed reading and enjoying the night rain. It reminded me of summers back home in Sweden. I was probably dozing because I made the first thunder-sound part of my dream. I thought I heard a car crash and sat up in bed with my heart pounding. I couldn't catch my breath or figure out whether it was night or morning. Then came the second clap of thunder and I said to myself, "Here I go again." All my life I have been terrified of thunder; my panic won't listen to logic. I ran around the apartment for no reason, and then pressed my fingers into my ears. It didn't help—I could still hear the thunder. Actually, waiting for each clap was worse than the noise itself. Thank God the storm passed quickly. When it was over, I laughed at myself; but I know the same thing will happen again and again.

For other women, phobias seem to emerge during a particular life phase and then disappear.

Leslie had never felt any anxiety about flying until her first child was born. Before that, she had always flown to and from Florida to see her grandparents and to vacation. She didn't anticipate her fear, but found that her first flight with the baby was torture. She listened to the airplane engines with terror, felt dizzy every time the plane hit an air pocket, and had ominous premonitions throughout the flight. The day before their return flight she felt nauseated, chilled, and terrified. She booked a train passage to New York instead, and found that her symptoms disappeared immediately.

For the next fifteen years, Leslie traveled by train or car, or chose not to travel at all. Although she knew that statistically air travel was safer than ground travel, she avoided flying at all costs. Even conversations with friends about vacations made her anxious. She tried not to make her fear of flying obvious, but her family and friends came to realize the enormous stress that she associated with flying.

In her late thirties, Leslie found that thinking about flying no longer made her upset. She joined her husband on a business trip, and was able to tolerate the flight with the help of a minor tranquilizer. She suspects that her phobia was related to her mothering role, but cannot explain its intensity or why flying was even more stressful than the inconveniences of not flying.

For yet other women, phobias have a strong symbolic meaning, although insight alone does not seem to free them of the phobia or its stress.

Selma is a high achiever who is unreasonably afraid of heights. She cannot take an elevator above the fourth floor of a building, will not look out of windows above jumping distance from the ground, and faints regularly if she must do so.

Her understanding of her phobia goes like this: "Being a success is very important to me. I am the oldest of four sisters and I want to maintain my lead in every way. I suspect that my fear of falling is like a fear of failure—losing my footing, losing my control. I'd rather walk up twenty floors of stairs than trust my life to an elevator. I'd rather miss a panoramic view than trust my safety to a guard rail. Sometimes it's a real problem because I have no choice in the matter. Then I suffer terribly!"

Psychologists disagree about the explanation of phobias. Many say they are responses produced by early classical conditioning—a type of learning by association. They mean that fear or anxiety has become automatically associated with a particular object or situation. Ingrid's fear of thunder, for example, they would assume was "learned" in this way many years ago. To unlearn this phobia, they would recommend counterconditioning. Thunderclaps would be paired again and again with pleasant images and relaxing circumstances until a new association had been formed. If these psychologists are right, Ingrid's thunder phobia would be gone and her stress level lowered. If they are wrong, however, the phobia would either reappear or a new symptom might take its place.

Actually, sometimes there is symptom substitution after counterconditioning, sometimes not. Perhaps there are several kinds of phobias. In addition to phobias learned through classical conditioning, there may be two other types. The first would provide a focus for what would otherwise be a sense of stress or anxiety too vague to get a handle on. Leslie's flying phobia would fit this model. Her concerns about mothering and the disasters that might befall her children become represented by flying. If she avoids flying, she feels as though she can avoid disaster and increase her sense of control.

The second type of phobia would express fear of an unacceptable impulse. Avoiding an object or situation helps to control that impulse. Selma, for example, may be frightened by an impulse to fall from her pedestal and give up her stressful high-achievement style. Avoiding heights gives her symbolic control.

Many phobias are less obvious than the three just described, even to the phobic woman herself. A woman may go through her day avoiding situations and objects without conscious awareness. She may label herself a procrastinator, forgetful, or harried. She may suffer much inconvenience and stress and still not admit to phobic functioning.

Here are some of the most common female phobias and their possible meanings.

PHOBIA	POSSIBLE FOCUS
Fear of crowds	Loss of identity
Fear of being alone	Learned helplessness/ dependency conflicts
Fear of being criticized	Good-girl complex
Test anxiety	Fear of failure/need for achievement conflict
Fear of injections	Concern about intrusiveness
Fear of small, closed places	Fear of being trapped or powerless
Fear of mice, snakes, spiders	Fear of loss of control

HIDDEN STRESS #6: GUILT

"Shoulds" and "shouldn'ts" both trigger guilt, and guilt is a powerful hidden stressor. Children struggle with "shouldn'ts" all day long. Women usually have very little time or opportunity to do things they "shouldn't" do—they struggle with "shoulds" instead.

> I should begin my diet today.
> I should finish the paperwork at my office.
> I should pay the bills today, but time flies.
> I should have called my mother-in-law, but I dread the conversation.
> I should bring the car in for a tune-up, but what an inconvenience!
> I should have gone to the PTA meeting, but they're so boring.
> I should spend more time with my son, but I am so busy.

I should be more patient with my boyfriend, but he acts like a kid most of the time.

Trying to be "good" is more frequently a source of stress for women than concern about being "bad." Trying to be a perfect daughter, wife, mother, employee, daughter-in-law, and friend, all at the same time, is often a female's fate. Girls are raised to be "good." They are praised and rewarded when they are empathetic, conforming, and considerate. Even when they enter the work world, they are expected to maintain their home responsibilities as well. Soon a pressure cooker of "shoulds" is building up steam. Result: the Female Stress Syndrome!

Eleanor set her alarm for six A.M. so that she could prepare the dinner she would serve her son and daughter-in-law that evening. It was her husband's birthday, and she felt that she should make it a special evening. Although she had not quite finished by seven, she knew she had to stop in order to straighten up the house before she left for work. Her husband awoke at 7:30 and rushed out, never noticing her secret preparations in the kitchen. She made the beds, dressed, and was out, herself, by 8:15 A.M.

The crosstown bus ran late and the subway was crowded. Eleanor stood all the way to the office and scolded herself for not leaving the house earlier. She arrived at work ten minutes late—a rare occurrence for Eleanor. Although nobody commented, Eleanor felt guilty. She skipped her lunch hour to get ahead on some work, but then realized that she should be more aware of her nutritional needs.

After work, Eleanor stopped at the bakery to

pick up a birthday cake she had ordered the day before. "I should have baked," she thought. "This is the first year in twenty-one years that I haven't baked, but I just don't have time since I started working!" Vague guilt gnawed at her as she rode home, standing all the way. She was tired, time-pressured, and dissatisfied with herself. She felt stressed, but the stress seemed unfocused.

Eleanor walked into the house and heard the sounds of the six o'clock news on the television. Her husband was both watching TV and reading a newspaper, while sipping a scotch and soda. As he rose to greet her, Eleanor heard herself snapping, "You know the kids are coming for dinner. Why are you acting like there's nothing to do around here?" He began to defend himself, but Eleanor accused him of starting a fight with her—and, indeed, got her fight.

It took Eleanor awhile to calm down and realize that she had been the one to start the fight, although to have admitted that she was using her husband to let off her own stress would have made her feel too guilty at the time. After all, it *was* his birthday!

The stress caused by guilt need not be as acute as that just described to affect a woman's day. If she anticipates criticism whenever she is less than perfect, she will always be ready for the worst. Checking the mail will be stressful—there might be a bounced-check notice, an insurance cancellation due to an oversight, or an unanticipated bill. Answering the telephone will be stressful, since the call may be from someone who is annoyed, requesting something, or complaining. Owing money takes on special meanings of inadequacy and embarrassment. A note from the boss or a child's teacher requesting a meeting becomes a notice of doom.

HIDDEN STRESS #7: LIFE EVENTS

Life events always involve stress. This is obvious if the event is an unexpected death, an unwanted divorce, or an incapacitating illness. It's less obvious if the event is a change for the good. But even good events, such as moving to a bigger house, changing to a better job, or having a long-awaited baby, can create stress by necessitating reorganization of time, energy, and expectations.

Test yourself on the Social Readjustment Scale of Life Events, developed by Thomas Holmes and Richard Rahe. Add up the indicated points for every life event or change that you have experienced over the past year.

SOCIAL READJUSTMENT RATING SCALE*

Life Event	*Point Value*
Death of spouse	100
Divorce	73
Marital separation	65
Jail term	63
Death of close family member	63
Personal injury or illness	53
Marriage	50
Fired at work	47
Marital reconciliation	45
Retirement	45
Change in health of family member	44

* Thomas H. Holmes and Richard H. Rahe, "The Social Readjustment Rating Scale," *Journal of Psychosomatic Research* 11 (1967), pp. 213–218.

Life Event	Point Value
Pregnancy	40
Sex difficulties	39
Gain of new family member	39
Business readjustment	39
Change in financial state	38
Death of close friend	37
Change to different line of work	36
Change in number of arguments with spouse	35
Mortgage over $10,000	31
Foreclosure of mortgage or loan	30
Change in responsibilities at work	29
Son or daughter leaving home	29
Trouble with in-laws	29
Outstanding personal achievement	28
Spouse begin or stop work	26
Begin or end school	26
Change in living conditions	25
Revision of personal habits	24
Trouble with boss	23
Change in work hours or conditions	20
Change in residence	20
Change in schools	20
Change in recreation	19
Change in church activities	19
Change in social activities	18
Mortgage or loan less than $10,000	17
Change in sleeping habits	16
Change in number of family get-togethers	15
Change in eating habits	15
Vacation	13
Christmas	12
Minor violations of the law	11

YOUR TOTAL: ____

In their sample poll in Seattle and from a Navy study of 2,500 subjects Holmes and Rahe found that people with scores over 300 points for one year had an 80 percent risk of becoming seriously ill or vulnerable to depression. Those with scores between 200 and 300 points still had an impressive 50 percent risk. Although these statistics cannot predict the risk for any particular individual, they do confirm the correlation between life-change stress and both physical and emotional health.

Now scan the Life Event Scale again. Note how many changes more frequently or more forcefully affect women than men: marriage, divorce, and reconciliation changes can totally restructure the daily life of a nonworking woman; son or daughter leaving home can trigger the "empty nest syndrome"; change in residence, recreation, church activities, social activities, family get-togethers, and the number of family members usually means more change for the wife than for the husband. Some life events are obvious, some are more subtle, but all contribute to the Female Stress Syndrome.

An examination of divorce stresses for women points up how important life changes are to female stress.

Stress begins long before the divorce, of course. During the decision-making process, a woman must typically consider problems most men do not. If there are children, in most cases they will reside with her after the divorce. If she is a working mother, she will have to do even more juggling, since she will then be breadwinner, mother, and sometimes surrogate father. Even if there are no children involved, her life-style will be drastically changed. She will give up her homemaker status for a round of dates and all the anxiety that involves: waiting to be called, battling the numbers that tell us there are more women than men available, competing with younger women for men of all ages, and being primarily reacted to on the basis of her appearance. Or perhaps she will give up companionship altogether, depriving herself of support. Furthermore, if she looks to romance or marriage as an important component of her happiness, she must deal with all of the above while shouldering a major disappointment, the failure of her marriage, freshly experienced.

Even for those women who wanted a divorce very much, stress will be produced by the life changes involved in the breakup. Their world becomes less predictable, and their future is again full of unknowns. According to William J. Goode in *Women in Divorce*, the most frequent symptoms of divorce stress among the 425 women he surveyed were

difficulty in sleeping	memory difficulties
poorer health	increased smoking
greater loneliness	increased drinking
low work efficiency	

Most interesting is the fact that he found the time of highest stress was the point of actual physical separation—the moving out—not, as he expected, the point of filing for divorce or getting the decree. Although the legal steps involve psychological changes, it is the process of moving out that most changes a woman's social status and relationships to her family and his, and has an impact on friends and children, on eating and sleeping patterns, on living arrangements, and so forth: life-change stress at its most intense.

MANAGING THE HIDDEN STRESSES

Step one in managing hidden stresses is to *uncover* the source of the stress. Many women are victims of guilt, phobias, impatience, noise pollution, driving anxiety, and hostess hardships without realizing that each continually contributes to the Female Stress Syndrome. Knowledge will not set you completely free, but it is a good start. The better you know yourself and your reactions to hidden stresses, the easier it will be to manage the stress and your reactions.

In most cases, a little reality-testing can go a long way. This is step two in hidden-stress management. It involves checking the old reaction against reality, and practicing a new, more appropriate response. Eleanor, for example, might try giving herself permission to revise her list of "shoulds," and might practice saying "It's OK" whenever she falls short of her own ideal. Selma might take herself by the hand and force herself to ride an elevator to the second floor of a familiar building the first week, to the third floor the next week, and so on.

Women suffering from a combination of noise pollution and a one-ear-always-listening-for-trouble syndrome may want to institute a "time of silence" policy, or hire a sitter to be the "listener" for an hour. Women who experience stress when they have to wait might carry a paperback novel, or a small notebook for doodling, making lists, and creative writing, or they might even practice the relaxation techniques discussed in Chapter 10 while on line at the bank.

Driving, of course, will always be somewhat stressful, although my patients have come up with many tension-reducers. One young mother plays symphonic music in the car. She finds that it is soothing to her and to her children as well. A commuter leaves a bottle of her favorite perfume in the car, her favorite chewing gum, and a set of cassettes that teach conversational French. She sprays the car with the perfume, starts chewing her gum, and practices her French all the way from Oakland to San Francisco! A more expensive tension-reducer is a CB radio. Listening to the verbal banter is fun; receiving traffic information is helpful; and knowing you have access to an emergency channel is reassuring.

Reducing life-change stresses requires using all the stress-management techniques you can muster. Since most life changes are either inevitable (such as the death of a spouse or a child leaving home) or generally irreversible (a divorce), stress management in these cases involves accepting the reality of the change. Replaying the past or pessimistically predicting a continuation in the future will not reduce stress. Addressing and dealing with the immediate present, however, will. As each step is taken, a sense of mastery and control will be gained.

Again, let's consider divorce as an example. Since your feelings about your ex-husband will change over time, don't worry now about a life of tense visitation episodes and never-ending squabbles over property or the "custody" of your best friends. If you have children who are negatively affected by the divorce, accept the fact that adjustment is part of growth and growth requires the passage of time. Do not assume that every problem of theirs that you observe can be directly attributed to the divorce or to your tension. Many of their problems are probably their *own*. Feeling guilty will not help you. Work with your children to master each problem day by day. You will all gain a greater sense of control. And finally, cancel whatever power you may have given your ex-husband to upset you. Listen to what he has to say to learn more about him and how he thinks, but don't collect his opinions about *you* to brood over in private!

The goal of hidden-stress management is to bring the stresses under greater control, reduce the feeling that you are being victimized, and modify stressed reactions. Change takes more than insight, however; it takes practice. Give it time, work at it steadily, and you will see results.

9

Female After Forty

Today, the average forty-year-old American woman can expect to live to be at least eighty years old. After the age of forty, then, many naturally start to re-examine their lives. Often they find they are as distressed as these women as they look into their future.

> "I used to think forty was middle-aged. Now that I *am* forty, I wonder if I was right."

> "My mother used to tell me: You live and learn. I have noticed that we live a lot faster than we learn!"

> "Marriage is a state of mind. I don't think I care for the mindless condition my marriage is in."

"Time seemed to go on and on until now. I thought that I had plenty of time to find a partner or husband, even to have a family. I may have waited too long."

"I used to think my work was everything. I no longer think *anything* is everything."

"Now that I am no longer needed by my children, I find that I don't want to be needed by my husband either. I suppose it's part of never having been free to be myself. I went from home, to marriage, to divorce, to marriage . . . without a breathing space. I don't want to divorce my husband, but I wish I had a *wife* for the next half of my life!"

"I am forty-five and still have not learned to relax. I don't know how to stop worrying about things I can't change."

"My children have grown up; my husband has regressed. He left me for a younger woman, and I am single, sixty, and sad."

"Just when I finished parenting my children, I had to start parenting my husband's parents. When do I get to take care of myself?"

"Going through menopause was like going through a rebirth for me. I began to think of sex as pure pleasure and looked forward to planning vacations without the kids. My husband, on the other hand, became depressed when he reached middle age, and I feel like I am living with an old man!"

> "I'm plagued by this nagging guilt now that my kids are out on their own. I'm so relieved not to have to worry about their food and clothing and schooling anymore. Does that mean I never really wanted to do it?"

"After forty, the crises never end," according to yet another woman. Bigger children have bigger problems, and then empty the nest. Husbands retire, leave, or die. Bodies sag, spirits flag, and backaches nag. Parents die and leave their children and children's children.

Unfortunately, it is during these middle years that many women experience more anxiety and depression than at any other life stage. Think of the many stresses produced by changing self-concepts, marriage dissatisfaction, redefinition of parenting roles, and the double standard of aging.

THE DOUBLE STANDARD OF AGING

In an article written more than ten years ago, Susan Sontag described the double standard of aging in this society by comparing older women and men. How much do you think has changed since she made these observations?

- As they grow older, women often keep their age a secret. Most men do not.
- Since women are often judged on their beauty and youthfulness, their value as partners may decrease as they mature. Since men are often judged on their competence and experience,

their value as partners may increase as they mature.

- As she ages, a woman's value in the job market-place often decreases, as does her pay. As a man ages, he can usually expect to be earning more than when he was younger.
- An older woman is considered less sexually attractive and desirable than a younger woman. An older man, particularly if he is financially or politically successful, does not lose his sexual eligibility. In fact, it often increases as his power increases, and the male/female mortality rates make him a scarce sexual commodity!
- Women experience menopause and, consequently, an anatomical and conceptual change of life; men may change their lives, but not through anatomical destiny.
- Older men can be expected to take younger lovers; older women are not!
- Women are expected to try to maintain facial beauty through cosmetics, moisturizers, and even surgery. Men are expected to have their faces become more rugged, scarred, and marked by the passing years.

Men and women do not approach the aging "starting line" neck and neck. Many of the stresses that affect women as they age have begun to form before they are forty. It is more often the woman than the man who has postponed or interrupted a career for the convenience of marriage or the necessities of parenting. It is more often the woman than the man who has assumed a submissive or compliant position when family decisions had to be made in the midst of pros and cons. It is more often the wife who is defined by her husband's status than the reverse. It is more often that a wife takes her husband's name than keeps her own—particularly among women currently over forty. It is not difficult to see the potential for stress in this sort of situation.

> Shirley flipped through the day's mail. There were eighteen envelopes. Fifteen were addressed to her husband. Two were addressed to "Resident." One letter was addressed to her. It was a note from her college alumnae association asking for a contribution to a scholarship fund. She looked again at this last envelope. In fact, it was not addressed to her at all. She had attended college under the name of Shirley Green, and this letter was addressed to Mrs. Richard Ashby. What has happened to Shirley Green? she wondered. She felt as though she had become some-bodys' mother, somebody's wife, and nobody at all to the outside world. By the time she was forty, she feared, she might disappear altogether.

Shirley did not disappear by the time she was forty. Instead, she wrote to her college alumnae association asking for her name to be listed as Shirley Green Ashby, took over the fund-raising division of the association in order to make sure other alumnae were similarly approached and addressed, and eventually formed a nonprofit organization that helps postgraduate women establish independent companies and develop self-employed careers.

Other women, unfortunately, see less-happy endings to their struggles to cope with the double standard of aging. Some lose their husbands to younger women. Some lose their dating momentum and settle for partners they would not have chosen a decade earlier. Some withdraw from the social or occupational spheres altogether, rather than risk losing out to other women. Some buy themselves cosmetic surgery and/or younger men. Whether we are married or single, no matter what our situation, the double standard of aging affects us and must be considered one of the special female stresses.

REENTRY AT FORTY

Many women who have spent the first two decades of their adult lives in the home see themselves as "just housewives," though this is an inaccurate and demeaning view. They complain that they lack job qualifications, social skills, sexual experience, and personal style. By the time they are approaching forty, they would like to reenter the world beyond their homes, but are stressed by what they consider their inadequacies.

Considering that the same activities they have performed are more valued when done by men than by women, low self-concepts among fortyish females are not surprising. Margaret Mead gives many examples of this phenomenon.

- Think of a woman cooking and you probably picture a housewife. Think of a man cooking and you picture a chef.
- Think of a woman working with clay, and you probably picture a craftsperson (or girl-scout leader, or kindergarten teacher). Think of a man working with clay and you picture an artist.

- Think of a woman assisting a childbirth, and you probably picture a nurse or midwife. Think of a man assisting a childbirth, and you picture an obstetrician.
- Think of a woman who is assertive. She is probably assumed to be aggressive. Think of a man who is assertive. He is assumed to be successful.

These generalizations help to explain why a woman with twenty years of homemaking experience often feels that she has little of value to offer in her later years. The reverse is true: A homemaker typically has experience in accounting, nutrition, paramedical activities, counseling, decorating, catering, social planning, and sometimes hiring, firing, and even public relations. If she has particularly enjoyed one of these areas, she can begin to focus her job or career ambitions.

In fact, the older woman is more desirable than her male counterpart both in the job market and as a mate. Research indicates that women have greater resistance to rheumatism, hemorrhages, many cancers, and brain disease. They usually have greater circulation of blood to the brain and suffer less loss of memory than men as they age. Since they retain the use of their hands, legs, and eyesight longer than men, women will remain occupationally and socially active longer.

Despite this positive report on women after forty, the myths often prevail. Husbands advise wives that they could not survive the "dog eat dog" world of business. Men tell women that their rages, hormones, or emotional temperaments make them too illogical to function well in a man's world. Even women often view other women with prejudices, and prefer to vote for male politicians, work for male bosses, hire male employees, use male lawyers, and choose male physicians!

SEXY AND SIXTY

The older woman is often more desirable than the older man in still another way—sexually. Although men have traditionally talked more about their sexuality, most women maintain their sexual interest and capacities far longer as they mature.

Excluding individual differences, medical problems, and situational factors, women in general experience fewer sexual problems caused by the aging process than men. Men find that their refractory period (the postejaculation phase of the sexual response when another erection is physiologically unlikely) increases with age and that partial or situational impotence becomes more common. With these problems frequently comes performance anxiety, which can inhibit desire and further interfere with male sexual functioning.

The older woman is in a different position. Menopause frees her from any pregnancy fears she might have had, and coincides with freedom from caring for small children and from her or her husband's career struggles. Menopause can replace premenstrual tension with hot flashes and other body changes, but hot flashes pass and other changes, such as diminished vaginal lubrication, can be treated medically or compensated for. The majority of women seem to adjust well physically to menopausal changes. Why, then, do we see female stress?

The main source of sexual stress among older women is older men.

Irene had been a bookkeeper for over twenty years, always looking forward to the time she and her husband would retire and move permanently to their country house in Maine. Her fantasy was that their time would be spent as their vacations there had been spent: gardening in the summer, reading, playing cards, and repairing in the winter, entertaining their children's children during holidays, and being close to each other. For Irene this meant romance. She and her husband had always been physically affectionate, cuddled, hugged, kissed, and found themselves making love with leisure and pleasure. Although she expected that the frequency of their lovemaking might diminish as they aged, she found her interest and enjoyment still held steady.

To her dismay, Irene foud that as the retirement date drew near, her husband drew away. He seemed less interested in both Irene and his own sexual pleasure. By the end of their first year in Maine, Irene and her husband were no longer making love. Disappointed and depressed, Irene tried to convince her husband to talk to a therapist. He refused. She eventually came to understand that her husband's loss of interest reflected both his loss of self-esteem when he retired from a responsible job and began to live on his wife's pension as well as his own income, and his expectation that to continue to be sexually active might stress his health. Perhaps, she speculated, intermittent intimacy was all her husband could handle emotionally. Being sexual as well as being together constantly would be too much for him.

Although their closeness and cuddling were restored, Irene and her husband did not share an active sex life in their later years. For Irene, this was a source of stress and frustration.

One point of this case history is that marriage itself does not insure that a sexually interested woman will have sex available in her later years.

Husbands may, for example, withdraw sexually after they have suffered a heart attack or other serious illness, even though their physicians have given them a go-ahead. The statistics on heart attacks, in fact, show a surprisingly low incidence rate of attacks during intercourse with a spouse. (It is slightly higher among men with new partners!)

Out of misguided concern, a man may also withdraw after his wife has suffered an illness. Psychologist Mildred Witkin of the Payne-Whitney Clinic has found that often a woman needs confirmation that she is still desirable after surgery, and waits for her partner to make the first move out of her own insecurity. Not surprisingly, Witkin found that the sooner women who have had breast surgery resumed their love lives, the more rapid and complete was their recovery from the psychological and physical effects of the operation. Indeed, this was a major factor in the recovery.

Husbands may withdraw sexually after high blood pressure medication, diabetes, or aging interferes with their erections. Most men do not know that they can have an orgasm with no erection at all. Furthermore, since women can enjoy all types of pleasuring and can have an orgasm from clitoral stimulation without intercourse, even total impotence does not have to mean an end to a couple's sexuality.

Husbands, finally, are often older than their wives. This is financially advantageous when a couple is young, but sexually disadvantageous when a couple matures. Add to that years of familiarity, routine, and daily problems. Add anxiety about appearance and performance. Add social taboos against "dirty old men." The result? Wives experiencing the Female Stress Syndrome!

Older women who are not married, or who never married, run the risk of additional problems in this area. Sexuality may be an inner quality, but sexiness, like beauty, is in the eye of the beholder. Without appreciative eyes around to behold you, it is all too easy to become lax about your exercise, diet, or appearance. Women over forty who are finding sexual partners less available should know that this is not so much a reaction against them personally, but rather the result of the double standard of aging as well as the unfortunate imbalance in the male/female populations in this age group.

The life expectancy for women in our society is still greater than that for men—six to eight years greater, on the average. By the time a woman is fifty, there will be approximately eighty men for every hundred women of the same age. By the time she is sixty, the number drops to seventy-two men per one hundred women; and after seventy-five, there are only about sixty-three men per one hundred women. Now consider that two-thirds of these men over sixty-five are still married; that leaves approximately one single man for every four single women over sixty!

Furthermore, as Susan Sontag noted, it is expected that men will date women their own age and younger. It is not expected that older women will do the same, even if they could. When an older woman is seen with a young lover, even today, most people assume that she is rich. These and other societal factors result in far fewer dating opportunities for older women than for older men.

STRESS AND THE NOT-SO-MERRY WIDOW

Another source of stress in the older woman is the experience of widowhood. There are now more than 10 million widows living in the United States, and, although women can of course be widowed at any age, they are on the average sixty-four years old.

When it comes to remarrying after the death of spouse, the odds are not in a woman's favor. Only one-quarter of all widows remarry within five years, compared to half of all widowers and three-quarters of divorced women.

Sheer loneliness is one of the biggest burdens of widowhood, whether it happens at a young or older age. H. Z. Lopata identified ten kinds of loneliness in widowhood that illustrate the stress experienced by many of these women:

missing the particular person
missing feeling loved
missing being able to love the other
missing an in-depth relationship
missing having someone else around the house
missing sharing work
missing the married life-style

missing the status of being escorted
increased strains on other relationships
difficulties meeting new friends

Compounding loneliness are ten additional sources of stress that have emerged from stress workshops I have run with widows.

1. Approximately 44 percent of widows must cope with a drop in their incomes when their spouses die. In addition, immediate funeral and other death costs average $4,000!

2. The majority of men die without leaving a will. This precipitates lengthy and confusing court procedures for their widows to handle.

3. Many widows can't escape the need to find an object of blame for their loss. They begin a litany of "if-onlys" that prolongs their mourning.

4. The woman who occupied a traditional role as a housewife usually suffers a sense of confusion and helplessness when the head of the household dies and she must take over.

5. Women whose husbands were financially and socially successful find both their status and feelings of security are diminished.

6. Depression in reaction to the death is often associated with early awakening and other sleep disturbances. These, in turn, reduce the widow's coping capacity and raise the risk of female stress symptoms.

7. If the widow's spoken communication is reduced with the loss of her husband, she may gradually withdraw from social contact. Such

withdrawal may become chronic, but it may not be obvious initially.

8. Many widows feel guilty if they find that they still have sexual needs. They feel disloyal to the deceased and inhibited about masturbation. Moreover, they are unlikely to find a suitable male partner. At present, two out of three women over sixty-five years in the United States are unmarried.

9. Widowhood is so common that it may not rally the social-support reaction it warrants. Since women tend to marry older men and then live longer than they do, for the most part, widowhood is epidemic! According to Metropolitan Life Insurance Company statistics, a woman's chance of widowhood is approximately 54 percent if her spouse is five years younger, 64 percent if her spouse is five years older, and 80 percent if her spouse is ten years older.

10. If a widow is forced by practical or financial circumstances to move after her husband's death, she must deal with the stresses of a significant change in routine, control, familiarity, and neighborhood support system. If, in addition, the change is to a child's home or to an old-age home, the loss of dignity and/or power and autonomy can be devastating!

AGING IN THE '80s

Although some of the stresses that beset women as they age are both universal and inevitable, others are unique to this time and place in history.

Women in the '80s are caught in the divorce deluge. Some women over forty are leaving their husbands; some are being left. Either way, more than 457,000 women forty or older were divorced by 1980. They have no models for their new life-style and no idea of what is to come. They are on the forefront of a new social world, caught in the stresses of changing expectations.

Women in the '80s are affected by the unique economic situation, in which inflation is coupled with a recession/depression. The golden years have become tarnished as pensions and incomes fall short of today's financial needs. Women worry about their own wage-earning capacities; about their retirement plans; about their security should they remain unmarried, or should their husbands die or leave; about medical costs; about their independence in their later years; and about their children's economic survival.

Women in the '80s are concerned about their daughters. Just as the lives of women over forty are radically different from the lives their mothers led, so are their own grown daughters' lives different. Their daughters are marrying later, working more, having fewer children, and divorcing more quickly. In *A Room of One's Own*, Virginia Woolf imagines the fate of an equally talented sister of William Shakespeare. As the story evolves, she is continually blocked from developing her talent by ridicule and prejudice. Today her fate might have been very different, but so might her stresses! With opportunity has come responsibility, choices, and risks. Today's women over forty do not escape the Female Stress Syndrome.

MANAGING AFTER-FORTY STRESS

Menopause

Perhaps more than at any other time in your life, your mind can make the difference in your experience of the Female Stress Syndrome after forty. Menopause, of course, is biologically programmed (unless surgery precipitates it), and the physical changes it brings are not totally under your control. But you can reduce the stress of feeling helpless and victimized by Mother Nature by maximizing your sense of *predictability*.

Women going through menopause should learn all they can about the changes they are experiencing. Learn that they are normal; learn that some have a limited duration; learn that they are not all mysteries; learn what changes will come next.

Although the menopause symptoms themselves may not be under your control, other areas of functioning are.

- Maintain control of your weight, following a nutritionally sound diet, and you will continue to enjoy your body.
- Set up and follow an exercise program. This will maintain your muscle strength and stimulate your energy supply.
- Schedule your time. Decide on your own priorities and handle time as if it were a very valuable commodity. Your time will truly be yours.
- Be good to yourself. This can help to reduce that feeling of being controlled by physical

changes rather than your own decisions. Treat yourself well: take bubble baths, read good books, eat delicious, nutritional food. Be as considerate of your own feelings as you are of others'.

- Take notice of your needs and be ready to *ask* for what may be needed from others: sympathy, support, closeness, distance, respect, or attention.

If the physical symptoms seem excessive, consult a gynecologist or endocrinologist.

If stress symptoms seem excessive, consult a psychologist or psychiatrist.

If you have a hard time deciding whether or not the symptoms are excessive, ask a professional that very question.

As previously mentioned toward the beginning of this book, there is a very positive side to menopause. Many women experience it as a relief, even as a rebirth. They find freedom from fear of pregnancy that is liberating both sexually and practically. With menopause comes a rite of passage into a period of personal choices and self-defined life-styles, free from premenstrual tensions and postpartum blues. With menopause often comes a reexamination of goals and roles, free from preparental anticipation and filled with postparental relaxation! Here at last is the opportunity to make resolves and choose courses of action that had been postponed, or not even considered. "It is time to get paid for my work," a mother of two college girls declared. "A job with pay will give me dignity and give my daughters a new way of thinking about me and themselves." And there are many women like Lena, who never considered that the years after mothering would be any less full or important, and planned for them.

Lena, now sixty-two years old, began planning for her eventual retirement from mothering when she was only thirty-eight. She started by enrolling in a counseling program that had evening classes, and by the time she reached menopause she had received her master's degree in social work. She had also completed her full-time mothering responsibilities. Lena feels that the fun has just begun since she started her private practice five years ago. She is pleased with the way she pursued her interests sequentially, rather than trying to juggle them simultaneously.

Managing the Stress of Grief

Although, of course, there are individual differences, widows may find comfort in the fact that grief and mourning often have distinct, predictable stages. Each is a necessary step in the natural healing process. Be aware of your own bereavement process and its stages. This awareness will not change your mourning, but will reassure you that your feelings are normal, and that mourning is a period that should gradually evolve into reengagement with the life around you. Milton Matz, a clinical psychologist and a former rabbi, has outlined the phases of bereavement.

Phase I: "If I deny it, it's not true"
The widow will try to avoid any thought or mention of the loss in an attempt to escape pain. This can be done in many ways. Some will act as if nothing had happened, for a while. They will attend to business and continue their work. Others will withdraw from

friends and family to avoid mention or association with memories of the deceased. Still others seem to be numb and unfeeling. Their lives and actions seem to be on automatic pilot.

Phase II: "I have the power to undo it"

During this stage, Matz suggests that many widows may try to escape the sadness of acceptance by utilizing magical thinking. Attempts to keep the spouse alive by "seeing" and "hearing" him are not uncommon, nor are beliefs that he is still right here on earth in spirit, to be communicated with. Women who have been raised to believe that women need men to survive daily life may try to undo the death of a spouse by immediately substituting someone—a son, a new spouse. Since the initial loss is not confronted, however, the mourning will continue and often interfere with new relationships.

Phase III: "I can't do anything about it"

The loss is faced and felt during this difficult period. The reality of the death of the spouse can lead to despair and even suicidal notions. The turning point will be not the acceptance of helplessness with regard to her husband's death, but power and control with regard to the widow's own *life*. As she makes choices and reshapes her life, reengagement will begin.

Phase IV: "I am rebuilding, and every now and then I remember"

According to Matz, there are as many reconstruction patterns as there are lives. In my clinical experience, I have noticed one common characteristic: the widow's healthy sense of surprise that she has been able to

manage her loss and grief, and often to feel stronger
for it. Widows realize that they were not merely half
of a pair, but are, in fact, a whole person in their
own right. Many choose to remain on their own and
enjoy the control they have over their lives.

If you have a friend who has lost her husband,
try helping her in the following ways:

- Allow her to formulate her own alternatives
  without overwhelming her with advice or threatening her sense of self-confidence.
- Do not deny her sorrow and loss. Reminding
  her that her spouse had "a good life" or died
  without pain will not address her personal separation anxiety, but, rather, may make her feel
  guilty for thinking of herself!
- Don't stay away. Although she may be withdrawn, upset, or proud, even silent company
  offers security.
- Offer social and work activities without pressure.
  Don't try to guess what is appropriate for her;
  everyone handles reengagement differently. Let
  her know that she is welcome to join life rather
  than being left to mimic death. It does not imply
  disrespect for her loss for her to function as fully
  as she can.

LIVING ALONE AND LIKING IT

If your marriage or long-term relationship ends, or you
have difficulty adjusting to the fact of being forty-plus
and on your own, there are a number of steps you can
take to make the experience more positive.

First of all, don't *judge* your needs. Don't stand back from yourself with your imaginary eyebrow raised and foot tapping while you assess whether you *should* need company. Instead, put yourself squarely on your own team and help yourself go after what you need to feel good without harsh self-judgments.

Turn to your family and friends. This is not a sign of weakness, not a lack of self-sufficiency. You're not the only one who needs to be needed. Think how good and useful it will make others feel to be able to give you pleasure or assistance.

Don't try to run away from intermittent sadness or loneliness. If you repress these feelings, the same repressive system will likely put the lid on *all* strong feelings—including joy and humor as well.

If a long-term relationship has just ended for whatever reason, accept the fact that you have gone through a transition and that any change, particularly one over which you have little or no control, will aggravate the symptoms of the Female Stress Syndrome. You may be more prone to depression or illness, depending on your "weak links." You may feel social stresses more, be more sensitive to insults and injuries from others. Remember that the Female Stress Syndrome is real—it's not all in your mind. Help yourself and be good to yourself.

If you have recently been widowed, be aware that guilt is a common side effect: guilt that you are still alive while your spouse is not, guilt that from time to time you felt anger toward him when he was alive, guilt that you may even be enjoying some aspects of your widowhood, guilt that feelings for another man may be developing.

Also, especially at first, take as much time as you can to make big decisions (such as whether or not to sell the house, where you should live if you do). If possible, don't let yourself be pressured into something before you're ready; in the midst of grief and coming to terms with a major life change, it is difficult to think clearly, and you may make decisions you will later regret. (One book dealing with this subject that you may want to consult is *Widow*, by Lynn Caine—see the Bibliography.)

Develop a network of people who share the same problems and feelings; you'll feel less alone. Fight some of the injustices of age prejudice, if that is your style. It will make you feel more potent. Keep in mind that as your sense of control increases, your stress decreases, so anything you can do to put yourself more in control of your life will go a long way toward easing the Female Stress Syndrome.

10

*Living with
Female Stress*

Up until now we have been examining the stresses that make up the Female Stress Syndrome, and the symptoms associated with those stresses. We have seen how the stresses that stem from a woman's biology and conditioning can trigger a wealth of physical and psychological ailments that, to one degree or another, are a fact of life for most of us. Now it is time to focus on *living with* the Female Stress Syndrome.

The aim of Female Stress Syndrome management is threefold. The first aim, which we have been discussing throughout this book, is to increase a sense of control. The higher one's sense of control, the lower one's stress. To take just one example, it has been shown that institutionalized, elderly people who are given certain choices—about which movie to see, which houseplant to own, which foods to eat—seem to cope much better, both physically and psychologically, than those who do not have such choices.

The second aim of Female Stress Syndrome management is to encourage realistic assessment of the stressful situation. Some stressful situations are short-term and require minor management efforts. Others are long-term and chronic—more likely to put women at high risk for stress symptoms, and requiring major stress-management efforts. Realistic assessment will not only help to distinguish between the two types of stressful situations, but will also help determine which are best handled through *action*, and which are best handled through *acceptance*.

The third aim of Female Stress Syndrome management is to improve problem-solving skills and coping strategies. Successful stress management should produce more than situational relief. Ideally, the process of managing stress should generate information on one's particular vulnerabilities and strengths, one's susceptibilities and capabilities. Every encounter with the Female Stress Syndrome should leave a woman better equipped to deal with stress when it next appears.

HELPING OTHERS

Everybody knows someone who is suffering from female stress and having difficulties managing it. It may be your mother, your sister, your daughter, your neighbor, your good friend. Fortunately, there is a great deal you can do to help her manage her Female

Stress Syndrome. The plan I recommend embodies many crisis-intervention techniques and family counseling approaches developed by psychologists throughout the past decade.

1. Look for the *"four D's."* They will let you know when a woman feels that she is in a crisis.

   Dependency needs are increased (though often denied!).

   Decision-making is difficult.

   Depression dominates the emotions.

   Disorganization and even panic sets in.

2. Show her that you *care*. Even if you share her alarm, do not show it—express concern instead. Try to understand the stress from her point of view, not your own. In this case the reality is not as important as the experience. Here are some things you might say.

   "I want to understand what you're going through."

   "I'm glad to have a chance to spend some time with you."

   "Have you ever gone through this kind of thing before?"

3. Encourage her to *talk* about her problem. Talking gives one a sense of "doing" something. Talking gives her an opportunity to "hear" herself, "listen" to herself as she would to another. Try saying:

   "Tell me a little more about this."

   "How do you explain that?"

   "I'm not clear about . . . "

   "What've you done that made you feel better (worse)?"

4. Be what psychologist Carl Rogers calls an *active listener*. Rogerian psychologists would recommend that you repeat what your friend or relative has said as a check for accuracy; repeat what you have heard to reassure her that you have really been listening. Repeat with warmth and sympathy to indicate that you accept the feelings being shared with you.

   "What I hear you saying is . . . "

   "I think I understand. You feel as if . . . "

   "You certainly seem to think . . . "

   "Do you mean . . . "

5. Help her to *help herself*. Taking over for her will only increase her sense of being overwhelmed, helpless, and out of control. Taking over will interfere with any learning that might otherwise result from managing a stress experience. To increase her self-help capabilities, follow the rest of the steps outlined.

6. Ask for a *plan of action*. Assess the risk-reward ratio. Discuss alternatives.

   "How do you plan to . . . "

   "What do *you* plan to do?"

   "Did you ever think that you might also try . . . "

7. Work on her *fine tuning*. That is, help her to focus on the problem without blurring the picture with exaggeration, anxiety, or anticipation. Sort the facts from the fictions.

   "From what you're telling me, it seems . . . "

   "Let me see if I can say that another way . . . "

   "What's the most practical way to go about this?"

"If you decide to do that, then you'll probably also have to . . . "

8. Develop a *contract* for a specific course of action. This accomplishes two stress-management goals. It makes her responsibility for
self-help clear, and it gives her a chance to
increase her self-esteem by carrying through
a plan during a stressful time.

"So by Wednesday, you're going to . . . "
"Now, I'm counting on you to . . . "

9. *Recapitulate* as often as necessary, since your
friend or relative is likely to be easily distracted.

"Now, you told me that you'd . . . "
"Let's make sure we know what we're
doing . . . "
"Tell me again what you're going to do
next."

10. Provide a *safety net*. Discourage withdrawal
from friends and family or support systems.
Encourage her to develop a network of re-
source people—informal "hot lines."

"Remember, I'll be around tonight at six and
tomorrow at . . . "
"Let's get together again tomorrow (Tues-
day, etc.) . . . "
"Who're you planning to spend the evening
(weekend, holiday, etc.) with?"

11. Set up *structure*. We all do better when we are
not at loose ends with time on our hands!
Mourning rites (wakes, shivas, etc.), baptisms,
confirmations, bar and bat mitzvahs, and even
weddings can provide structure during periods

of transition or stress. Make use of such social institutions.

12. There are cases in which we are dealing with a problem that cannot be truly "solved" (one-sided love, fatal or chronic illness, etc.). In these cases, promote appropriate *acceptance*. This will help reduce useless persistance and directionless activity; and it will help reduce the effects of the Female Stress Syndrome.

HELPING YOURSELF

Always remember, as I said at the outset of this book, that *you are entitled to try to reduce the stress in your life.* Give yourself permission to take control over your life, to stop feeling guilty, to worry less about the "shoulds" that inevitably crop up.

Separate Your Past from Your Present

Don't re-create old scenarios again and again with the new people in your life. They will not change in the reliving. They will not give you mastery over the past. Instead, address the present: it is the present over which you can really take control.

Don't assume the future will be the same as the past. Our view of the past is never objective anyway. Our earliest introduction to the world leaves a lasting impression, it is true; however, this first impression can be sorted out from the more complex reality of the present. The child's view in each of us can be recognized by us, tolerated with self-affection, and then redirected and guided by the adult in us.

Accept Yourself as a Package Deal

You cannot be perfect. Don't even try. Instead, as I recommended before, aim at being able to describe yourself accurately. As you allow yourself to be a less-than-perfect package, you will allow others to be so also. As you begin to describe rather than evaluate yourself and others, your stress level will go down. Replace "This is who I should be" with "This is who I seem to be." Work with your reality, not your ideal. This is vital to managing the Female Stress Syndrome.

Break the Habit of Living Life Laced with Guilt

When we are young, most of our guilt follows behavior that we learned was *bad*. When we are adults, however, we have little time or impulse to be "bad." More often, our guilt follows behavior that falls short of what we learned was *good*. Women say to themselves "I should have . . ." all day long.

"I should have said yes . . ."
"I should have said no . . ."
"I should have called . . ."
"I should have offered . . ."

This type of guilt serves no purpose except to increase stress. It is after the fact and therefore cannot be helpful. Replace self-recrimination with self-observation.

"It seems I did not want to say yes . . ."
"I wonder why I did that . . ."
"Would I prefer, next time, to . . ."

Learn to Say No

Learn to say no without feeling guilt (as to a child).

Learn to say no without justifying yourself (as to your spouse).

Learn to say no without defending yourself (as to a parent).

Learn to say no graciously, not tentatively (as to your lover).

Learn to give explanations, not excuses (as to the boss).

Give Yourself the Freedom to Change Your Mind

Don't persecute yourself every time you change your mind about something or someone. Reassessing is a mark of flexibility, not instability. Although a "whim of iron" may represent too much mind-changing, a happy medium is better than rigid, inappropriate consistency.

Become Your Own Permission-Giver

You don't need permission from others to take care of yourself, to reduce your own stress level. Don't wait until the whole world can see that you are under stress before you allow yourself a rest. Don't wait until you feel you can't cope with one more problem before you start to take care of yourself. If you wait for others to take care of you, you might wait forever. Even if no one else in your life recognizes the reality of the Female Stress Syndrome, by now you do.

Give yourself permission to

- Rest: take a nap, a bath, or whatever—you're entitled!
- Relax: read a book, watch television, write a poem, listen to music, nap—and don't *contaminate* this relaxation time with chores.
- Set realistic limits: underwhelm yourself, underschedule yourself, and underdemand—don't worry, I'm sure you'll find that you still have too much to do!

Become Your Own Best Friend

Be on the lookout for stressors that trigger your stress symptoms. Protect yourself as you would your other loved ones.

Become Your Own Resource Person

Learn how to manage *emergencies* that are inevitable or highly probable: funeral arrangements, medical crises, auto disasters. Compile lists of hot lines, professionals, and references.

Learn how to manage your reactions to those *situational stresses* that particularly affect you: holidays, in-law problems, or financial worries. Don't be caught upset; anticipate and alleviate your reactions.

Learn to manage *chronic stress* in order to protect yourself from serious Female Stress Syndrome symptoms. Pay attention to the factors that make such situations better or easier for you—and the factors that make them worse.

Become Your Own Catharsis Expert

For short-term or emergency stress, catharsis techniques can help you cope. Catharsis is the emotional equivalent of a pressure cooker blowing off some of its steam through the lid valve. If the valve becomes stuck and the pressure builds to the point of eruption —pot roast on the ceiling! Catharsis techniques aim at discharging the tension that accumulates during stressful situations. They increase our sense of control by giving us the means to moderate our pressure levels, vital during times of stress. They exercise and relax our bodies, make good use of the extra adrenaline produced during stress, and direct "nervous" energy. They provide a healthy distraction from our immediate stress.

Some cathartic activities are self-regulated and self-contained. They don't require a partner or equipment. They include

- Walking—The most common exercise for both men and women of all ages.
- Calisthenics—About 17 percent of men and women twenty to forty-four years of age work out at home or in health clubs.
- Swimming—15 percent of women surveyed report that they find swimming very relaxing.
- Jogging—Fast becoming the most popular stress antidote!

Other cathartic activities are competitive. They include

- Tennis
- Racquet ball, paddle ball
- Team sports
- Marathons
- Games (backgammon, cards)

Become Your Own Relaxation Expert

Counteract tension with a soothing environment. Warm baths, hot tubs, long showers, Jacuzzis, whirlpools, saunas, and steam rooms all work for some women. An hour in a library, museum, gallery, bookstore, or favorite chair with a book or music help others.

Stanley Fisher, a New York psychologist who specializes in teaching autohypnosis for relief from pain, phobias, and presurgical anxiety, among other stress-related problems, recommends that you use autohypnosis to let your body know that this is its time to relax. The simple steps for entering and exiting from autohypnosis are as follows.

1. Sit comfortably in a chair facing a wall about eight feet away. Pick a spot or an object on the wall that is about one foot above your sitting eye level. This is your focal point.
2. Look at your focal point, and begin counting backward from 100, one number for each breath you exhale.
3. As you count and continue to concentrate on your focal point, imagine yourself floating, floating down, down through the chair, very relaxed.
4. As you stare at your focal point you will find that your eyelids feel heavier and begin to

blink. When this happens, just let your eyes slowly close.

5. While your eyes are closed continue to count backward, one number for each time you exhale. As you count, imagine how it would feel to be as limp as a rag doll, totally relaxed and floating in a safe, comfortable space. This is your space.

6. As that safe, comfortable feeling flows over you, you can stop counting and just float.

7. If any disturbing thought enters your space, just let it flow out again; continue to feel safe and relaxed.

8. When you're ready to come out of autohypnosis, either let yourself drift off to sleep, or count from one to three and exit using the following steps. At *one*, let yourself get ready; at *two*, take a deep breath and hold it for a few seconds; and at *three* exhale and open your eyes slowly. As you open your eyes, continue to hold on to that relaxed, comfortable feeling.

You can also counteract tension with progressive relaxation. Some of my patients make a tape of their own voice issuing the following instructions:

1. Starting with your toes, relax them.
2. Then the feet and ankles: relax.
3. Then the calves: relax.
4. The knees: relax.
5. The thighs: relax.
6. The buttocks: relax.
7. The abdomen and stomach: relax.
8. The back and shoulders: relax.

9. The hands: relax.
10. The forearms: relax.
11. The upper arms: relax.
12. The neck: relax.
13. The face: relax.
14. Drift off.

Finally, try counteracting tension with the following technique. You will first slowly contract and relax each part of your body for ten seconds each; and then contract and relax each part of your body more quickly to become aware of the tension-relaxation contrast.

1. Frown as hard as you can for ten seconds; then relax those forehead muscles for ten seconds. Now repeat this more quickly, frowning and relaxing for one second each and becoming aware of the different feelings of each movement.
2. Squeeze your eyes shut for ten seconds, then relax for ten seconds. Repeat quickly.
3. Wrinkle your nose hard for ten seconds; then relax for ten seconds. Repeat quickly.
4. Slowly press your lips together; then relax. Repeat quickly.
5. Press your head back against the wall, floor, or bed (real or imaginary)—then relax. Repeat quickly.
6. Bring your left shoulder up in a tight shrugging motion; relax. Repeat quickly.
7. Do the same with your right shoulder; repeat quickly.

8. Press your straightened arms back against the wall, or floor, or bed; relax. Repeat quickly.
9. Clench your fists tightly for ten seconds. Relax your hands and let the tension flow out through your fingers. Repeat quickly.
10. Contract your chest cavity for ten seconds and release. Repeat quickly.
11. Press your back against the wall or floor; relax. Repeat quickly.
12. Tighten your buttock muscles for ten seconds; relax. Repeat quickly.
13. Press your straightened legs against the wall or floor or bed; relax. Repeat quickly.
14. Slowly flex your feet, stretching your toes as far back toward you as possible; relax and let tension flow out through your toes. Repeat quickly.
15. Check for tense spots and repeat the exercise where you find any.

Soon you will begin to recognize muscle contractions caused by tension before these contractions can cause spasms and chronic pain.

Create Self-Fulfilling Prophecies

Expect the best. Even if things do not work out the way you might have wanted them to, at least you have not stressed yourself *before* the problem or disappointment. In other words, reduce *anticipatory anxiety*, which does not change outcomes but only increases the risk of the Female Stress Syndrome.

Use the "as if" technique. That is, behave *as if*

everyone would be delighted to treat you just the way you want to be treated.

> Rosalie was meeting her friend David for dinner. She very much wanted to attend a party for city singles later on in the evening, but worried that David might be insulted if she tried to socialize with other men, or angry if she added another activity to their plans. She decided, however, to put the "as if" technique to work before abandoning the singles' party idea. After all, she reminded herself, she and David were "just friends," not lovers.
>
> Rosalie presented the party plan to David as if she expected him to be delighted and appreciative. "Guess what," she began. "After dinner, I've arranged it so that I can take you with me to the best singles' party in town. We can compare notes when it's over. Aren't you lucky to have me as a friend?" Indeed, David responded by agreeing.

Similarly,

> Ellen was trying to attend a college in the evening and run a three-child household at the same time. She needed her husband's moral support, financial aid, and household help. She was feeling that she wasn't entitled to them, however. "Going to college is so self-indulgent," she thought. "I really should be working part time, rather than studying part time," she chided herself. Although her husband had not said a word against her studies, she was always prepared for his criticism. She read things into his remarks, became defensive if he was tired, and felt angry if he wanted her time. She put herself under so much pressure with this anticipatory anxiety that she was ready to quit college.

As a last resort, Ellen decided to try the "as if" technique. She gave herself permission to be a part-time student and began to behave as if she believed it was fine with her husband, too. Now she was able to react to his helpfulness with appreciation rather than guilt, and she never let an opportunity go by to praise his support in front of friends.

In Ellen's case, the "as if" assumption was closer to reality than her own pessimistic assumptions. Her husband increased his efforts to be helpful and understanding, and she felt less stressed.

The "as if" technique, as I have suggested before,

- Facilitates asking for favors without a trace of defensiveness.
- Facilitates asking for favors without the flavor of anticipatory anger.
- "Teaches" others that we see ourselves as worth positive treatment and entitled to consideration.
- Flatters others by making *requests* of them—not demands.
- Reinforces reactions in others that will reduce, rather than increase, stress.

Remember, don't sabotage your own communications by broadcasting expectations of disappointment, or by broadcasting criticism.

Enjoy Your Own Sexuality

If you have a sexual partner, don't neglect the sexual side of yourself when you are under stress. For many women, sexual activity is an important outlet for tension. It helps women remember that they are desirable, attractive, needed, or wanted. And by being intimate, they close out the rest of the world temporarily, providing a vital respite from stress.

If you are orgasmic, your sexual experience will leave you relaxed due to the role of the parasympathetic nerves in orgasm. The capacity to masturbate, therefore, is also very important as a stress reliever.

Stay Self-Centered

By self-centered I do not mean selfish; I mean self-aware. Remind yourself continually to look at yourself and at the world through your *own* eyes, not through others' eyes. Looking at yourself through others' eyes is called "spectatoring," and it can raise performance anxiety, which is a component of the Female Stress Syndrome. If you suffer from shyness, self-consciousness, and lack of spontaneity, spectatoring is probably your problem.

Do not constantly view yourself through others' eyes and change your opinion of yourself and of your decisions, even when important people in your life disagree. Don't reevaluate yourself every time your partner, children, or friends disapprove. Don't give others the power to knock you off balance. Stay centered.

Assess Your Stress

You cannot manage stressors or symptoms until you can identify them. With pencil in hand, review the list of stress symptoms on page 193. Add others in the blanks provided. During the course of a day, note the time when you experienced any symptom on the list. Next to the time, jot down the activity you were engaged in or about to begin. Do you find a pattern?

TIME	ACTIVITY	SYMPTOM
		Headache
		Heartburn
		Nausea
		Cold sweat
		Dizziness
		Memory block
		Asthma
		Hyperventilation
		Allergic reaction
		Backache
		Swallowing difficulty
		Rapid heartbeat
		Increased blood pressure
		Urinary frequency

If you find that certain activities seem to trigger stress symptoms for you, deal with them in the following ways:

1. Assess the timing of the activity. Could you do the task earlier or later in the day? Would this make a difference in terms of stress?
2. Assess your performance level. Are you over-invested in this activity? Are you spending too much time and energy in this area?
3. Assess your motivation. Are you letting a sense of "should" dictate your behavior? Too often an activity we might enjoy is resented because we feel compelled rather than motivated to complete it.

Anticipate the Stress of Holidays

Don't feel guilty or surprised if holidays are stressful. Everyone finds them so. Holidays involve a change in schedule, a gathering of family, and high expectations —usually too high! For many, they evoke upsetting memories of good times lost or bad times past. For some, they emphasize feelings of being alone and isolated. Holidays can also encourage regression to childlike feelings without childhood's satisfactions. And most people find that holidays require extraordinary preparation, work, and cleanup. Don't be fooled by the fantasy that everyone else's Christmas is warm and wonderful. Some are, of course; most aren't.

Take holidays one moment at a time. Some moments will be memorable; some will be disappointing. Enjoy what each *does* bring: food, a break from work, visual beauty, religious feelings. Try not to compare a holiday experience with those past, or with those to come.

Aim for Self-Management, Not Quick Change

As we noted before, your personality structure was years and years in the making. Your earliest years constituted your introduction to "reality." Because those years preceded speech, they are not even accessible through your memory. Think back to your earliest memory. Chances are you are thinking about something that happened when you were two or three years old. Your sense of safety, security, and self had long since begun to form. Think back to your twelve years in grade school. Can you remember every teacher you had? No? And yet you spent a *year* with each!

Restructuring a personality would obviously take as long as the five most formative years and then some. Although psychoanalysis attempts this, most stress reduction can be more quickly and realistically achieved by *knowing* your personality structure than by changing it. Work *with* your defenses, strengths, and weaknesses, not against them. Self-deprecation increases stress; self-management does not. Unrealistic attempts at personality change are frustrating and increase stress. Self-acceptance does not.

Move Into the Here and Now

Many women increase their stress by being so pulled into reliving past problems and so pushed into "preliving" future fears that they are rarely living in what gestalt psychologist Fritz Perls called the "here and now." Life is literally passing them by, and so are opportunities for quiet moments, little pleasures, and deep breaths. If this is one of your problems, continually bring yourself back from upsetting hypothetical scenarios into the present, and try to live life as an ongoing process, not a series of upcoming crises.

Practice, Practice, Practice

Therapists have learned that insight is usually not enough to change behavior. What is needed after insight is practice, practice, practice. Practicing new behaviors leads to new types of reactions from others, new information about alternatives, and new views of realities. Start practicing now.

When you are under stress, practice *acting*, not reacting.

1. Help yourself do this by taking the time to collect information about a situation or person before you draw conclusions. If someone's behavior is upsetting, don't take it personally. Process what you are seeing and feeling as information, not insult. Decide how *you* feel about what they are saying or doing, and what their behavior says about them.

2. Help yourself do this by determining the logical consequences of the situation or of someone's behavior, not by dwelling on illogical "what ifs," or "This must mean that . . ." Check out all assumptions you are making before acting on them.

3. Help yourself by *not* giving others the power to

make you react before you are ready. Take your time.

4. Help yourself conquer spectatoring by practicing placing your focus on others as you interact, not on yourself. If someone's reaction threatens to throw you off balance, practice staying centered. Mary Beth does this when she is confronted by saying: "I understand your point and I will think about it." Laurie tells her friends: "I find what you say very interesting." Paula just says: "Hmmmmmmmmmm!" when she feels stressed and ready to react defensively.

5. Help yourself by recognizing when you are backing off from a goal because of fear of failure, rather than moving forward toward it. Remember the ring-toss study? Practice focusing on the stake. Walk right up to your goals; don't back off. Since you will try to achieve your goals anyway, why make your job harder by handicapping yourself?

Laugh, Laugh, Laugh

Laughter is the signal for the Female Stress Syndrome centers to turn off the emergency adaptation system. As Norman Cousins suggests in his book *Anatomy of an Illness*, laughter may even promote healing. What a delightful tool for stress management! It defuses tension when an embarrassing topic has come up in a joke, when an unacceptable thought or impulse has been spoken out loud, or when a perspective has been changed or regained. It lights up our faces, relaxes our muscles, lowers our sense of vigilance, restores our objectivity, and enhances hope.

Pursue Both Short-Term and Long-Term Remedies

As you begin to develop your own stress-management program, keep in mind that you will need to continually pursue both short-term *and* long-term remedies. Exercise, autohypnosis, relaxation techniques, sex, and even laughter are short-term remedies that will help you feel more comfortable with your body and more positive about yourself. They provide immediate gratification and release. Long-term solutions, including the various aspects of behavior modification discussed in this chapter—learning to live in the present rather than in the past, learning to feel less guilt, accepting what you cannot change about your life, giving yourself permission to take time off and reduce stress—will increase your sense of control and help reduce chronic stress. Both kinds of techniques are vital to counteracting the stress in your life.

The stresses that plague women are a part of our lives; so too are its symptoms. We cannot ignore them, feel guilty about them, or let them overwhelm us. Recognizing the effect they have on us means that we will no longer need to turn to others for an incomplete explanation of what is going on. Learning how to manage them means we will no longer need to settle for the recommendation that we simply get a good night's sleep—or take two Valium. Female stress must be taken seriously—by women, their families, and their friends. It must be countered with understanding, self-help, and, where appropriate, with professional help.

Turn your hand palm-up and look at what is called your lifeline—the line that starts between the thumb and first finger and curves around the base of the thumb almost to the wrist. Your lifeline has a beginning, a middle, and an end. It does not go on forever. Life, too, has a beginning, a middle, and an end; it, too, does not go on forever. From now on, whenever you look at your hand, be reminded that the time to reduce stress is *now*! Don't wait until stress symptoms overwhelm your capacity for work or play. Don't wait until your doctor, family, or friends beg you to start taking care of yourself.

I began this book with a quotation from Hans Selye: "Complete freedom from stress is death." Contrary to public opinion, he points out, we cannot avoid stress. We are in fact *surrounded* by stress, especially where money, work, family, children, and sex are concerned. We experience stresses connected with our physiology, stresses hidden in our daily routines, and stresses that crop up at holidays and even on vacations. Short-term stress can help us achieve what we want to achieve. Long-term stress can help us mature—but only if we gain control over it where possible and, where it is beyond our control, try to manage the effects it has on us. More than ever, it is vitally important that we learn how to live with stress, so that we can really enjoy the full, healthy lives we were meant to have.

Bibliography

ABERLE, D., and NAEGELE, K. "Middle Class Fathers' Occupational Role and Attitudes toward Children." *American Journal of Orthopsychiatry* 22 (2) (1952): 366–378.

ABRAMSON, M., and TORGHELE, J. R. "Weight, Temperature Change, and Psychosomatic Symptomology." *American Journal of Obstetrics and Gynecology* 81 (1961): 223–232.

BARRY, H.; BACON, M.; and CHILD, I. L. "A Cross-Cultural Survey of Some Sex Differences in Socialization." *Journal of Abnormal and Social Psychology* 55 (1957): 327–332.

BARUCH, GRACE K., and BARNETT, ROSALIND C. "Implications and Applications of Recent Research on Feminine Development." *Psychiatry* 38 (1975): 318–327.

BLOCK, J. H. "Conceptions of Sex Role: Some Cross-Cultural and Longitudinal Perspectives." *American Psychologist* 28 (1973): 512–526.

BREIT, ETTA BENDER, and FERRANDINO, MARILYN MYER-

SON. "Social Dimensions of the Menstrual Taboo." In *Psychology of Women*, edited by J. Williams. New York: W. W. Norton, 1979.

BRYSON, R. B., et al. "The Professional Pair: Husband and Wife." *American Psychologist* 31 (1976): 10–16.

BUDOFF, PENNY WISE. *No More Hot Flashes and Other Good News*. New York: G. P. Putnam's Sons, 1983.

CAINE, LYNN. *Widow*. New York: Bantam Books, 1975.

COLEMAN, J. C. *Psychology and Effective Behavior*. Glenview, Ill.: Scott, Foresman & Co., 1969.

COSTRICH, N.; FEINSTEIN, J.; and KIDDER, L. "When Stereotypes Hurt." *Journal of Experimental and Social Psychology* 11 (1975): 520–530.

COUSINS, NORMAN. *Anatomy of an Illness as Perceived by the Patient*. New York: W. W. Norton, 1979.

DALTON, KATHARINA. *The Premenstrual Syndrome*. Springfield, Ill.: Charles C. Thomas, 1964.

DOHRENWEND, B., and DOHRENWEND, B. "Sex Differences and Psychiatric Disorders." *American Journal of Sociology* 81 (1976): 1447–1454.

DOUVAN, ELIZABETH. "The Role of Models in Women's Professional Development." *Psychology of Women Quarterly* 1 (1976): 5–20.

EDELMAN, BARBARA. "Binge Eating in Normal Weight and Overweight Individuals." *Psychological Reports* 49 (1981): 739–746.

FREEDMAN, ALFRED; KAPLAN, HAROLD; and SADOCH, BENJAMIN. *Modern Synopsis of Comprehensive Textbook of Psychiatry/II*. Baltimore: Williams & Wilkins, 1978.

FRIEDAN, BETTY. *The Second Stage*. New York: Summit, 1981.

FRIEDMAN, MEYER. "Type A Behavior: A Progress Report." *The Sciences* 20 (2) (1980).

FRIEDMAN, MEYER, and ROSENMAN, RAY. *Type A Behavior and Your Heart*. New York: Alfred A. Knopf, 1974.

GOODE, WILLIAM J. *Women in Divorce*. New York: The Free Press, 1956.

HOLMES, D. S., and JORGENSEN, B. W. "Do Personality and Social Psychologists Study Men More than Women?" *Representative Research in Social Psychology* 2 (1971): 71–76.

HOLMES, T. H., and MASUDA, M. "Psychosomatic Syndrome." *Psychology Today*, April 1972, 71–72.

HOLMES, T. H., and RAHE, R. H. "The Social Readjustment Rating Scale." *Journal of Psychosomatic Research* 11 (1967): 213–218.

HORNEY, KAREN. *Feminine Psychology*. New York: W. W. Norton, 1973.

KAPLAN, HELEN SINGER. *The New Sex Therapy*. New York: Brunner/Mazel, 1974.

LAMANNA, MARY ANN, and RIEDMAN, AGNES. *Marriages and Families*. Belmont, Ca.: Wadsworth, 1981.

LEVI, LENNART. "Environmental Factors in Stress and Coping." *Stress and Coping*, Report No. 3. Philadelphia: Smith, Kline & French, 1981.

LEWIS, MICHAEL. "Early Sex Differences in the Human: Studies of Socio-Economic Development." *Archives of Sexual Behavior* 4 (1975): 329–335.

LOPATA, H. Z. "Loneliness: Forms and Components." *Social Problems* 17 (1969): 248–261.

LOPICCOLO, J., and LOPICCOLO, L., eds. *Handbook of Sex Therapy*. New York: Plenum Publishing Corp., 1978.

LUETGERT, M. J., et al. "Today's Feminist: Her Place is in the Home!" Paper presented at meeting of American Psychological Association, Chicago, Ill., 1975.

Bibliography

McClintock, M. K. "Menstrual Synchrony and Suppression." *Nature* 229 (1971): 244–245.

Maccoby, Eleanor E. "Sex Differences in Intellectual Functioning." In *The Development of Sex Differences*. Stanford, Calif.: Stanford University Press, 1966.

Maccoby, Eleanor E., and Jacklin, C. *The Psychology of Sex Differences*. Stanford, Calif.: Stanford University Press, 1974.

McGuiness, Diane. Quoted in "Just How the Sexes Differ," by D. Gleman et. al. *Newsweek*, May 18, 1981, 72–74.

McKinlay, S., and Jeffreys, M. "The Menstrual Syndrome." *British Journal of Preventive and Social Medicine* 28 (2) (1974): 108.

Masters, William H., and Johnson, Virginia E. *Human Sexual Inadequacy*. Boston: Little, Brown & Co., 1970.

Mead, Margaret. "On Freud's View of Female Psychology." In *Women and Analysis*, edited by Jean Strouse. New York: Grossman, 1974.

Meyer, J., and Sobieszek, B. "Effect of a Child's Sex on Adult Interpretations of Its Behavior." *Developmental Psychology* 6 (1972): 42–48.

Money, John, and Ehrhardt, Anke A. *Man and Woman: Boy and Girl*. Baltimore: Johns Hopkins University Press, 1972.

Paige, Karen. "Effects of Oral Contraception on Affective Fluctuations Associated with the Menstrual Cycle." *Psychosomatic Medicine* 33 (1971): 515–537.

Parlee, Mary Brown. "The Premenstrual Syndrome." *Psychological Bulletin* 80 (1975): 454–465.

PERLS, F., HEFFERLINE, R., and GOODMAN, P. *Gestalt Therapy*. New York: Delta, 1965.

PRIBRAM, KARL. Quoted in "Just How the Sexes Differ," by D. Gleman et. al. *Newsweek*, May 18, 1981, 72–74.

PUNER, M. "Will You Still Love Me?" *Human Behavior* 3 (1974): 42–48.

REBELSKY, F., and HANKS, C. "Fathers' Verbal Interaction with Infants in the First Three Months of Life." *Child Development* 42 (1971): 63–68.

REES, L. "Premenstrual Tension Syndrome and Its Treatment." *British Medical Journal* 1 (1953): 1014–1016.

ROGERS, CARL. *Client-Centered Therapy*. Boston: Houghton Mifflin, 1951.

RUBIN, J.; PROVENZANO, F.; and LURIA, Z. "The Eye of the Beholder: Parents' Views on Sex of Newborns." *American Journal of Orthopsychiatry* 44 (1974): 4.

SCHMALE, A. H., and IKER, H. P. "The Effect of Hopelessness and the Development of Cancer." *Psychosomatic Medicine* 28 (1966): 714–721.

SEARS, R.; MACCOBY, E.; and LEVIN, H. *Patterns of Child Rearing*. Evanston, Ill.: Row, Peterson, 1957.

SELYE, HANS. *The Stress of Life*, rev. ed. New York: McGraw-Hill, 1976.

————. *Stress Without Distress*. New York: Signet, 1974.

SERBIN, LISA A., and O'LEARY, K. DANIEL. "How Nursery Schools Teach Girls to Shut Up." *Psychology Today*, December 1975, 56–58.

SHERMAN, J. A. *On The Psychology of Sex Differences: A Survey of Empirical Studies*. Springfield, Ill.: Charles C. Thomas, 1971.

————. "Social Values, Femininity, and the Development of Female Competence." *Journal of Social Issues* 32 (1976): 181–195.

SONTAG, SUSAN. "The Double Standard of Aging." *Saturday Review*, September 23, 1972, 29–38.

SPEROFF, L.; GLASS, R. H.; and KASE, N. G. *Clinical Gynecologic Endocrinology and Infertility*. Baltimore: Williams & Wilkins, 1973.

STAFFORD, R.; BACKMAN, E.; and DIBONA, P. "The Division of Labor Among Cohabiting and Married Couples." *Journal of Marriage and the Family* 39 (January, 1977): 43–57.

TASCH, R. "The Role of the Father in the Family." *Journal of Experimental Education* 20 (1952): 19–61.

TELLER, SANDY. *This Was Sex*. Secaucus, N.J.: Citadel Press, 1978.

U.S. BUREAU OF THE CENSUS, Statistical Abstract of the United States: Washington, D.C., 1981.

WILLIAMS, JUANITA H. *Psychology of Women*. New York: W. W. Norton, 1977.

WILLIAMS, JUANITA H., ed. *Psychology of Women, Selected Readings*. New York: W. W. Norton, 1979.

WOLBERG, L. R. "Hypnotic Experiments in Psychosomatic Medicine." *Psychosomatic Medicine* 9 (1947): 332–342.

WOLMAN, BENJAMIN B. *Handbook of General Psychology*. Englewood Cliffs, N.J.: Prentice-Hall, 1973.

WOLPE, J., and LAZARUS, A. A. *Behavior Therapy Techniques: A Guide to the Treatment of Neuroses*. New York: Pergamon Press, 1968.

WOOLF, VIRGINIA. *A Room of One's Own*. New York: Harcourt, Brace & World, 1929.

Index